Lynda Birke is biologist
surrounding gender and
Feminism and Biology (1986,
and *Their Problems* (Virago
Through the Microscope (Virago ... *han the Parts:*
Biology and Politics (1984). She lives in Buckinghamshire.

Susan Himmelweit teaches economics and women's studies at the Open University. She was a founder member of *Feminist Review* and has been involved in several campaigns around reproductive rights. She has written extensively on the political economy of women and the place of reproduction in society. She lives in London.

Gail Vines is a science journalist especially interested in genetics and in making science accessible to women. She is currently features editor of the *New Scientist* magazine. She lives in Buckinghamshire.

The first 'test-tube' babies are now adolescents. Yet at the mere mention of in vitro fertilisation, surrogate mothering or prenatal diagnosis, arguments rage. What is the controversy really about? Should research on embryos be permitted? Should fetuses carrying genetic diseases be aborted? Are women's rights of paramount and overriding importance? Much feminist writing on the subject expresses a complete rejection of reproductive technologies based on fear: fear that we are witnessing a takeover by scientists of women's reproductive role. The authors recognise the origin of this fear but do not agree with the conclusion. They argue that technological solutions are not always bad for women: and women have to be informed if they are to make choices.

Tomorrow's Child tells you how these technologies work and how they are likely to develop; it discusses the ethical dilemmas, and the assumptions made about fetuses and women; and above all it contributes to the debate by suggesting strategies by which women can take control.

Tomorrow's Child

Reproductive Technologies in the 90s

Lynda Birke
Susan Himmelweit
Gail Vines

Parts of Chapter One have been adapted
from an article that originally appeared
in Feminist Review, No. 29, Spring 1988.

Published by VIRAGO PRESS Limited 1990
20–23 Mandela Street, Camden Town, London NW1 0HQ

Copyright © 1990 Lynda Birke, Susan Himmelweit and Gail Vines

All rights reserved

A CIP catalogue record for this book
is available from the British Library

Printed by Cox and Wyman Ltd, Reading, Berks

To the memory of
Hilde Himmelweit
who always believed that
sense would triumph in the end

Contents

Preface and Acknowledgements ix

Introduction 1

Part 1

1. Reproductive Freedom, Technology and Society 13

2. Science, Technology and Nature: Women's Friends or Foes? 43

3. The Medicalisation of Reproduction: Justifications and Assumptions 60

Part 2

4. What Goes Wrong? Reproductive Technologies and Infertility 77

5. Fertilisation and IVF 103

6. What Can Go Wrong? Implantation and Pregnancy 130

7. Detecting Genetic Diseases: Prenatal Screening and its Problems 157

Part 3

8. Towards a Reproductive Future?   205

9. Official Attitudes to Reproductive Technologies in Britain and Elsewhere   232

Conclusion: Policy and Politics   282

Notes   317

Index   337

Preface

There have been many books in the last decade about the 'new reproductive technologies'. So why write another? Most previous books fall into one of three types. First, there are books written by the 'experts' outlining the wonders of modern science and what it can do for people experiencing reproductive problems. These books do not question the technology or the practices of the scientists who create them. Nor do they always tell women everything they might want to know, for example, about the dangers of particular techniques.

A second kind of book deals with the ethical questions. Should research on human embryos be permitted? What should be done with 'spare' embryos, fertilised in vitro but no longer needed by the women for whom they were created? Should fetuses carrying genetic diseases be aborted – or do such fetuses have a right to be born? And so on. These questions tend to be concerned with the rights of embryos, fetuses and new-born babies. What is generally lacking from the books that deal with such ethical issues is any consideration of the rights of women, the people who will not only bear the children, but also the brunt of the problems that may ensue in raising them.

A third category of literature does take women's rights and needs to be paramount. Over the last few years, feminists have paid increasing attention to developments in reproductive technologies. Much of this writing expresses fear: fear that what we are witnessing is a takeover by scientists of women's role in reproduction, and fear that we are moving towards a dehumanised (and defeminised) technological future. The position such books adopt is one of total resistance to scientific and male control of reproductive processes, by a complete rejection of the new technologies.

We recognise the origins of that fear; but we do not agree with the conclusion. One reason we do not is that it comes into conflict with one of the main principles for which feminists have fought, that women should be able to choose whether or not to bear a child. Although it has its limitations, the rallying cry of the struggle over abortion, that it should always be a woman's right to choose, remains for us central to developing a feminist politics of reproduction. If women want to try technological solutions to their reproductive problems, we may be unhappy about the risks they could be taking with their own health; if women want to avoid bearing children suffering from a particular disease, we may have fears about the implications for society. But we feel that women, and women alone, should be the ones to make the choice. That still leaves room for us to hold views as to how we hope those choices will go, to enter debate on the issues raised and to struggle to make the conditions under which reproductive choices are made less constraining.

But in order to make choices, women have to be informed. And if women are to participate in discussions about reproductive technologies, to have a say both in the future direction of research and how it is currently used, then it is essential to know what is going on, to understand what the scientists are trying to do and how far they have succeeded. So in writing this book we wanted to be as informative as possible about what is happening in the development of new reproductive technologies – at least up until the time of writing; this field changes rapidly. At the same time we have explored the ethical problems debated by others, in so far as we have considered them relevant to women. And we have also added our own particular feminist voice to the debate about how women should respond to the technologies; a voice that may sound more rational than polemical and seem perhaps to be lacking some of the passion of feminist writings which reject reproductive technologies out of hand. If it sounds this way, then this is because of our commitment to women forming their own opinions and making their own choices, both about their own lives and the political positions they hold, not because we do not care about the outcome.

This book, then, is a particular amalgam of all three approaches we mentioned above. It is partly about the science itself, describing what happens in particular techniques such as in vitro fertilisation. It is partly about the ethical dilemmas, and the assumptions these make about fetuses and about women. And it is partly about feminist resistance to others, be they scientists, clergymen, lawyers or politicians, taking control of women's reproductive lives. Above all, we hope it is a contribution to women taking such control themselves.

Acknowledgements

Many women have helped us to think in general about the role of reproduction in society and women's relationship to science and technology, both of which are crucial underlying concerns of this book. We have also benefited from talking to a number of women in various countries about their views on new reproductive technologies. We would particularly like to thank the women who took the time and trouble to read and comment on all or part of the manuscript, even if we have not always followed their suggestions: Alice Henry, Hilde Himmelweit, Anne Phillips, Ruth Wallsgrove and an anonymous reader for the publisher.

Introduction

In October 1979, 50,000 people marched through the streets of London in support of abortion rights. The march was organised by the Trades Union Congress around the slogan 'A Woman's Right to Choose' and marked the first time anywhere in the world that a trade union federation had taken up the fight for abortion. It attracted wide support from male as well as female trade unionists and, at the same time, criticism from some feminists who saw the trade union movement as muscling in and trying to take over a struggle about an exclusively women's issue.

Nevertheless, that the march was held at all was remarkable. Until shortly before then, Labour Party Conference had repeatedly refused to support abortion rights for women on the grounds that it could not pass binding resolutions on what had to be a moral issue of conscience for individual MPs to decide. But in 1975, and again in 1977, the conference decided to support women's rights to abortion and this has gradually become accepted as Labour Party policy, though not one that has been effectively enforced. The defeat, so far, of all bills aiming directly or indirectly to restrict the 1967 Abortion Act has been the major, perhaps the only, parliamentary success for women since Margaret Thatcher became prime minister.

A survey conducted in 1979 by National Opinion Polls showed that 56 per cent of the population agreed and only

29 per cent disagreed with the proposition that 'abortion should be made legally available for all who want it'[1]. This proposition went far beyond existing legislation, which made abortion legal subject to two doctors' assessment of a woman's reasons for wanting a termination, rather than giving the woman alone the right to decide. It appeared that a woman's right to choose not to bear a child had been won, morally in the minds of the people, even if the law had not yet recognised it in practice.

But even as abortion rights were being won, black women were urging caution. For them, the issues concerning reproductive rights turned more often on the right to bear children in the face of pressure for contraception, abortion and sterilisation. Institutionalised racism had led to black fertility being treated as a problem in itself, making the apparent goal of the population planners and even of some doctors to reduce the birth-rate of black babies, rather than to enable black women to have control over their own fertility. And what appeared to be true about attitudes to black women in this country was even more apparent when applied to whole populations of non-white women. For example, injectable contraceptives, whose side effects were considered unacceptable for white women, were advocated with enthusiasm for third world women. To the population controllers the main advantage of these contraceptives was that once injected they required no action by the woman herself, and were therefore more 'effective' than those that gave women the opportunity to exercise control.

To encompass such a range of problems and abuses surrounding reproduction, the feminist concept of 'reproductive rights' was created. This was to include both the traditional focus of feminist campaigns on abortion and contraception, the right of women not to reproduce – and to be treated as more than just reproducers – and the right of women to reproduce and to control the circumstances under which they do so.

The women's movement in other countries recognised the

need for such a broader focus on reproductive rights earlier than in Britain. In the United States, the Committee for Abortion Rights and Against Sterilisation Abuse has called for improvements in childcare provision at the same time as challenging attempts by the 'moral majority' to restrict abortion rights and reintroduce forced sterilisations. The International Contraception, Abortion and Sterilisation Campaign, and its successor, the Women's Global Network on Reproductive Rights, has made the fight against forced sterilisation and for the provision of maternal and infant health care as important, on a world scale, as campaigning for access to safe abortion and contraception. In Britain, the National Abortion Campaign split in 1983 on the question of whether it should continue to be a single-issue campaign. Those that favoured a wider reproductive rights focus set up the Women's Reproductive Rights Campaign, to campaign on a wide variety of reproductive issues including reproductive hazards at work, safety controls on contraception and improved availability of NHS abortions[2]. The Women's Reproductive Rights Information Centre was set up simultaneously to provide women with information on a wide range of reproductive matters such as methods of contraception, pregnancy testing, access to abortion, prevention of infertility and methods of treatment. It has since become the Women's Health and Reproductive Rights Information Centre, expanding its range to include women's health care in general as well as continuing to provide information on campaigns throughout the world on reproductive rights and women's health issues[3].

Feminism has changed in other ways over the past couple of decades. In the early 1970s, when the current wave of feminism began, most of the women involved in the movement either had had their children and were searching for other means of fulfilment in their lives, or had not had children and were not yet having to face the issue of whether they ever would choose to be mothers. Both groups saw it important to prove that women did not have to be seen only in terms of their reproductive abilities. For both groups, reproductive freedom meant freedom *from* reproduction.

But since then, some of these same women have become more interested in the possibility of having children. Partly this has been a matter of ageing; women who were in their early twenties in 1970 are by now facing the fact that even delayed childbearing cannot be delayed forever; women approaching forty cannot avoid the question of whether to have children, though they do not have to give the expected answer. But it has also resulted from a changed political climate, which has affected younger feminists too; feminism is no longer for many women the totally absorbing activity and form of self-definition it once was. Feminists, like others, may be turning inwards to rear children, perhaps as the only social contribution to make in a period of reaction and political quiescence, rather like the way the American left reared a whole generation of 'red diaper' babies during the McCarthy years, who later grew up to join the anti-war movement of the 1960s. Babies themselves, not just the limitations they impose on their mothers' lives, have, after a period of near oblivion, become a matter of interest to the women's movement. And this has led a few feminists to experience problems with their own fertility, and even more to take an interest in the issues surrounding pregnancy and childbirth, including infertility and its treatment.

Although some forms of treatment for infertility have been available in the past and the women's health movement has always stressed preventive care, it has been the advent of what are called the 'new' reproductive technologies that has rather belatedly put such issues onto the feminist agenda. It is partly the success of previous campaigns that has been responsible. For, as the availability and acceptability of abortion has grown, the number of babies put up for adoption each year in Britain and throughout the developed world has fallen dramatically, effectively closing off, for most people, one traditional solution to involuntary childlessness. This has focused attention on solutions that attempt to overcome directly the effects of infertility itself, by enabling such women to conceive and/or bear a child themselves. The traditional methods of infertility treatment, involving lengthy investigations, unglamorous operations to unblock tubes, low-tech mechanical devices or drug treatment, have not excited attention. Rather, it is the newer, flashier technologies of conception which, despite their low success rates and failure to treat the underlying infertility, have hit the headlines and left a trail of unanswered political questions in their wake.

Not all new reproductive technologies are aimed at the infertile, helping them to bear a child if they want to. Another set are designed to help people to have a healthy 'normal' child, by allowing a range of congenital defects to be detected prenatally. The availability of abortion has been central to the opening up of these technologies too, for the only 'cure' for nearly all such detectable defects is abortion, although methods of treatment in the womb for some fetal handicaps are promised for the future. Controversy surrounding such attempts to help women to bear a normal child turns not only on the ethics of whether a fetus found to be suffering from a congenital defect should be aborted – and if so what range of defects merit such treatment – but also on what the effects on society as a whole would be if parents were able to specify characteristics of the child they were to have.

The issues raised by these technologies are not all new – indeed some of the technologies themselves are not so very new. But they have now been raised in a more concentrated and explicitly political form, which forces their attention upon us – in arguments about the personal, private nature of our reproductive decisions, about our attitude to nature and its control, about the dangers of large and expensive technology and the lack of access women have to it. Should individuals be free to choose whatever reproductive strategies they like, whatever the consequences for society of a mass of individuals making similar choices? And what do we mean by free choice for women over reproduction anyway, in a world in which we have been taught to see ourselves primarily as wives and mothers? And what of the future? If we accept these technologies now because they may help a few infertile women to bear children or prevent a few babies with crippling diseases being born today, may they be developed and used in much more sinister directions in the future?

New reproductive technologies have gathered a wide range of opponents, from some feminists who fear that women may lose what little control they currently have over their reproductive abilities to their reactionary opponents who fear precisely the opposite, that women shirking their traditional reproductive responsibilities will lead to a breakdown of family values and the benefits of civilisation as we know it. The technologies also have their equally enthusiastic supporters, among them the practitioners and researchers themselves, who fear that opposition may prevent them from perfecting their techniques to help the infertile and hold back the growth of scientific understanding. And, of course, there is an increasing number of women who have chosen, for one reason or another, to use reproductive technology. Among them, besides a much larger number of disappointed ones whom the technology has failed to help, are some infertile women who have succeeded in giving birth to children they never thought they would have, and other women who have been spared the sadness of giving birth to a child with a congenital disease, but instead had to face the trauma of a late abortion.

On abortion, feminists have, in general, had little difficulty agreeing a political position, one which insists that all women should have access to safe abortions, and that they and they alone should be the ones to decide whether to have an abortion or continue with a pregnancy. Such a political demand could have taken many forms, but in practice, it has tended to be focused around individual rights, with the phrase 'A Woman's Right to Choose' becoming universally recognised as referring to abortion. There have been problems with this approach: too little recognition that the question of freedom of choice has to be seen within the context of societal constraints upon that choice and too little attention paid to the actual availability of abortions, for example. But in general the reproductive rights focus has been quite successful, relying as it does on an idea that is generally approved of in Western societies: that individual people should be free to make their own decisions about matters concerning their private lives.

New reproductive technologies also raise the question of reproductive choice, but they raise a whole number of other issues about women's position in society that go far beyond the question of individual rights. This is not surprising; the negative freedom not to bear a child, which access to abortion guarantees, is undoubtedly less complex than its obverse, and to some people more questionable right, the 'right' to bear a child. Indeed it may well be that the relatively immediate and individualistic position of a 'Woman's Right to Choose' needs reworking if a consistent feminist position on women's reproductive rights in general is to be developed. For it is an illusion to think that the issues surrounding the 'old' reproductive technologies, such as abortion, are any simpler in reality. They also raise questions about women's access and control of technology and the alternatives to motherhood available to women in our society. Abortion, even if it were really available on demand, would offer women only the 'choice' between bearing or not bearing a child under current social constraints. Economic and social circumstances can be just as powerful a factor forcing a woman not to bear a child as a law forbidding abortion can be in forcing her to bear one; the large number of women willing to undergo illegal and dangerous abortions before the 1967 Act is sufficient evidence of that. A position based on an individual's right to choose might have appeared to be adequate when talking about a woman's right to sufficient control over her own body not to have to go through an unwanted pregnancy or give birth to an unwanted child; but its inadequacy becomes clear as soon as we consider what a feminist position should be on the circumstances in which women positively wish to bear children.

For beyond the question of the right to choose, there are also questions concerning the significance of motherhood in our society, what children mean to all of us and the social circumstances in which we raise them. Recent feminism has largely been based on demonstrating that women can do other things besides bearing and raising children. New reproductive technologies for overcoming infertility, however, show that some women are prepared to go to remarkable lengths to have children. This has been cited as evidence by feminism's critics of an underlying, and biologically determined, maternal drive that feminism has failed to shift. On the other hand, it can also be seen as a demonstration of the strength in our society of a maternal ideology that insists that women have to have children to be fulfilled, an ideology that feminism still has to combat. With this in mind, some feminists have suggested that, rather than encouraging an infertile woman to turn to such technological solutions, the problem of infertility should be seen more as one of living in a society that gives a woman no positive image of herself other than as a mother. Recognising this, what should our attitude be to the technologies that seem to offer hope to such women? Are infertile women helped by being able to resort to reproductive technologies, or does their existence – and the promise they unreliably offer – merely intensify the ideology of motherhood? These questions and others about the social circumstances within which reproductive technologies must be assessed will be discussed in the next chapter.

Chapter Two looks at another set of issues surrounding new reproductive technologies; those to do with science, in particular the biological and medical sciences. This chapter will examine some of the approaches feminists and others have taken to science and technology. It will also explore how science has seen us, and what this means for the way in which scientists and doctors treat women and especially women in their reproductive roles. New reproductive technologies have generated a great deal of fear about the directions science can take, what might happen to an area of our life if scientists take control, what indeed scientists' aims are and whether we can influence these and shape science in ways that help women.

In the first two introductory chapters, we shall be looking at the questions new reproductive technologies raise at their most general level, without examining the particular technologies to which they apply. But since the technologies are significantly different from each other, the issues surrounding them differ too. For that reason, later chapters of this book will discuss the specific questions raised by each type of technology. These chapters of the book, however, are structured not so much around the technologies but around the biological processes in which they intervene. Each chapter describes a particular stage in the normal, that is unassisted, process of reproduction. It then discusses what can go wrong at that stage, the technological possibilities of intervention and the controversies surrounding them.

After discussing today's technologies and the controversies to which they give rise, we shall go into a more speculative realm and talk about the future. Some feminists are worried about current reproductive technologies not so much because of the way they are used now, but because of fears about the way in which they, or more powerful technologies yet to be developed, might get used in the future. We discuss such future scenarios in Chapter Eight, as well as considering what further technological developments we can realistically expect in the near future and some of the issues to which these might give rise.

Chapter Nine looks at the history of controversies surrounding reproductive technologies and examines the official view embodied in the Warnock Report[4], the enquiry set up by the British government in 1982 to consider the social implications of new and potential developments in reproductive technology. In doing so, some of the underlying issues surrounding attitudes for and against particular practices will be drawn out with a view, in the final chapter, to making some recommendations about how feminists might respond to the challenges posed by new reproductive technologies.

Part 1

1. Reproductive Freedom, Technology and Society

Deciding whether or not to have a child is one of the most important decisions a woman can make. The decision to have a child may be part of a rational plan, may be taken only as a result of an unplanned pregnancy, or may, indeed, not be a willing decision at all, but something forced upon a woman. However it comes about, having a child means an abrupt and important change in the way a woman lives her life; she becomes a mother, with all the expectations, obligations and pleasures associated with that role in current society. Similarly, not to have a child, though this may evolve as an eventual outcome rather than be the result of a decision actively taken, is also a major step for a woman. In taking it, and thereby rejecting society's expectations of her as well as both the work and the rewards of the social institution of motherhood, she sets herself apart from the lifestyle of the majority of her contemporaries. For good or ill, her life is also structured by that decision.

Because reproductive decisions take on such significance, not being able to carry them out, through a denied abortion or through infertility, for example, is a serious problem for many women. All reproductive decisions can be taken only within the context of society, which means that the decision either way is heavily influenced by economic pressures, the expectations put on women and the alternatives society leaves open to them. This means that the problems of not being able to carry out one's wishes about reproduction also have to be seen within the context of society and the pressures within it on women to have children. In order to examine debates surrounding new reproductive technologies it is therefore necessary to examine how and why women in our society make the decision to become mothers.

Why Do Women Become Mothers?

There has been a long-standing argument between feminism and its critics as to why most women choose to have children and how such a choice should be treated. However, although this debate has been going on for some time and the questions it raises are fundamental to feminism, new reproductive technologies have given such questions a directly political edge. Feminism has always been committed to giving women a real choice as to whether they wish to fulfil the traditional role of motherhood, by being positive about alternative lifestyles and images of women. If reproductive 'rights' are to be extended to apply to women involuntarily infertile, then their choice to bear children has to be seen as equally authentic. But can this really be the case in a society which insists so strongly that women have to be mothers in order to be fulfilled?

For a long time, modern feminism consistently defended any woman's right not to bear children but was much more ambivalent about a woman's desire for children. This led opponents to claim that feminists are anti-children and that in bringing child-bearing into question they are trying to persuade women to defy their natural instincts. These 'biological determinists' represent the desire of a woman to bear a child at its crudest as a purely natural, biological instinct. Such instincts are genetically programmed into all living creatures, for without them their genes would die out and, in the language of modern genetics, survival and transmission of one's genes is what life is all about. For men this is relatively straightforward; the best way to propagate their genes is to impregnate as many women as possible and hope that a few will survive. For a woman, however, a better way to ensure the transmission of her genes is to make sure that the small number of offspring that she is physiologically able to bear grow to maturity. This 'socio'-biological account of why women want to bear and raise children mirrors, in the roles it assigns to parents, the sexual division of labour and sexism of our society. It takes no account of anthropological data which show that the roles of men and women vary across different societies. Instead, it is a theory which seeks to universalise and 'explain' the particular habits of this society by claiming that women's desires in all societies are determined by their reproductive biology, that all women in this are the same and that therefore all women want to have their own children[1].

According to most feminist critiques this is ethnocentric nonsense. Of course, biology enters into the construction of all of us and may well affect our desires. But this cannot be the end of the story. Our lives are not determined purely by biology; indeed, one of the specific biological characteristics of human beings is that they are able to adapt to different environments and in turn shape those environments. In other words, by changing the circumstances in which we live we change ourselves. It is that ability to adapt both themselves and their environment that has allowed human beings to survive in a variety of relatively hostile settings. The elaborate construction that is modern society is a product of precisely that sort of adaptation. People have made society but people are also moulded by society, so that no aspect of their behaviour or desires can be purely natural, nor, on the other hand, can any aspect be purely social.

In Britain today, the vast majority of women have children. Indeed, by the time they had reached the age of forty, 90 per cent of women born in 1945 had had children[2]. This figure has not always been so high[3]; in other periods of history as many as one third of women may not have borne children. And today some women have actively chosen not to have children, either because they do not particularly care for them or because they prefer to do other things with their lives. There are, however, strong social reasons why most women do end up having children at some point in their lives. These reasons can be explored at a number of different levels.

First, there are the economic and social pressures on women to marry and become mothers. For many women today, and for most women in the past, marriage can be explained in purely economic terms, even if other factors are usually present. Women's wages are consistently lower than men's; a woman's main chance of having access to the benefits of the wage only a man can earn has always been to marry one. Today, we tend not to see marriage in such mercenary terms, but until quite recently that would not have been so shocking. And even today, when young girls dream of their future in terms of marriage and a family, it is a married lifestyle in all its material reality that they are thinking of, which inevitably compares unfavourably with the less affluent conditions in which most single women live.

And children are part of marriage; the wife's traditional role within the family is to provide and look after the children, a role she still fulfils even if she also goes out to work. If we choose to look at it in purely economic terms, the children are her meal-ticket and her occupation: both her means of escape, whether real or imagined, from a boring badly paid job and what keeps her from thinking of herself in terms of a career and acquiring the skills needed for more fulfilling employment. And, until recently, children were an inevitable part of marriage – for the fertile. The social and economic expectation placed on most women is that they will become mothers, and this expectation has in turn frequently prevented even those who will not have children from exploring and realising other opportunities in their lives. The effect of expectations like these works not only on the economic level. Girls who are brought up to expect to be mothers can feel they have failed if they do not fulfil those expectations. The considerable training for motherhood they acquire as girls is not just a set of skills; it includes feelings about what they should do with their lives: both positive feelings about their abilities to mother and, often, negative feelings about their chances of success and fulfilment in the world outside motherhood. So even those women who have the economic means of 'escape' from maternity often do not take them; they still want to be mothers, as well as or instead of participating in the public world of employment. Indeed, the difficulties of combining childcare with a worthwhile career often result in women jeopardising themselves economically in favour of motherhood.

In this way, parents provide role-models for their children which in turn the children live to recreate and provide similar models for their children; for women, this means that little girls learn to fulfil their mother's role. Psychoanalytic accounts have criticised this rather simplistic view of how we learn to become mothers and have more theorised versions of how the desire to mother is reproduced. The traditional Freudian view is that women can resolve early experiences of loss and incompleteness only by having a child, and that these experiences are the result of realising that they, like their mother, do not have a penis. But this view has been criticised by feminists as, effectively, a form of biological determinism itself. Instead, feminist psychoanalysis has talked about such feelings of loss and the consequent need for a child to mother being reproduced in girls by the experience of having someone of the same sex as themselves as their primary caretaker, their mother, an experience a boy does not have[4]. In this version then, the specific social arrangements for raising children that we have today, of the nuclear family within which mothers do most of the childcare, are marshalled to explain women's desire for children. Again, the habits of society are seen to be as important as biology, if not more so, in explaining why women want to have children.

Many specialists working on new reproductive technologies seem to consider the desire of the infertile women they treat for children as strong, natural instincts which do not need to be explained. As a consequence, they believe their work should be seen as unquestionably beneficial, for only good can come of helping such women to fulfil their natural instincts. In contrast, most feminists believe that the maternal desires that such women hope new reproductive technologies can fulfil for them are by no means uncomplicated, natural desires. Indeed, some feminists would argue, they are precisely the socially produced needs that have been most detrimental to women. According to this view then infertility is a problem for women only because they live in a society which encourages women to see themselves as nothing more than potential mothers. It is the failure of women to view themselves as anything more than potential mothers that leads to their wish to use reproductive technologies to fulfil a particular limited vision of themselves. Rather than encouraging women to do so, we should work to transform society in such a way that women do not feel they have to be mothers.

Both attitudes, those of the specialists and their feminist critics, seem to imply that socially produced desires and needs are in some sense not quite as real as some other more 'natural' ones. The doctors put an importance on fulfilling desires they think of as natural, that they would not accord to wishes they thought were less natural, such as a desire by men to be given hormones to allow them to breastfeed, for example. Feminists who argue against the use of reproductive technology for infertile women, however, may in some cases be adopting a similar attitude by refusing to recognise the importance of the wishes of such women to be mothers. Acknowledging the extent to which such desires are socially conditioned seems by itself to reduce their importance, as though the moment the artificiality of feelings is recognised they can be overcome. The reality, as many feminists – including those who themselves have faced infertility problems – have discovered, is not so simple. Understanding where a need comes from does not remove it. Nor indeed is there any difference in the desire for children from any other in that respect. All needs and desires are socially produced, whether or not, like feelings about reproduction, they centre on a process that has some biological content too.

On the other hand, feminists who consider the strength of maternal ideology to be irresistible and infertile women so 'desperate' that they are incapable of making choices about their treatment, fall into the opposite trap of overestimating the power of socially produced needs. Some argue that the medical profession succeeds in entrapping women into their programmes because effectively brainwashed infertile women will do anything to have children[5]. Their views, conversely, also have something in common with the belief of some medical specialists in an inescapable maternal instinct which similarly makes infertile women prepared to try anything to fulfil their desperate need for children. There may be strong pressure, from ideology or even from instincts, on women to be mothers in our society, but we are all subject to pressure in many areas of our lives and that does not make us incapable of making choices or the decisions that we take any less worthy of respect.

Given the difficulty of changing individual desires, there have to be strong arguments about the social undesirability of a practice if it is not to be employed to try to satisfy such desires. We have to be careful not to load onto the infertile (or, similarly, onto those who might have to bear the problems of raising a handicapped child) any greater demands of self-sacrifice in the interests of society than we require of those whose reproductive lives prove less problematic. If motherhood is a trap for the infertile, at least those who decide to go for treatment have actively chosen it; they are likely to have considered its pitfalls more carefully than women who never had any trouble conceiving. Having fought for fertile women to be able to decide these important matters for themselves, we should not then hold a much more patronising attitude to infertile women and see them as incapable of making choices. Nevertheless, the possibility of treatment for infertility may, in practice, further intensify the pressure on women to see themselves as incomplete unless they are mothers. If the existence of new reproductive technologies and the 'hope' that they bring, unmatched by success rates, undermines women's confidence in themselves as anything other than mothers, then reproductive 'freedom' for women may be diminished rather than increased by their existence.

The Question of Choice

Most feminists have supported 'A Woman's Right to Choose' on abortion while recognising that choice always takes place under constraints and that women can never have real reproductive freedom in a society in which they are subordinated. Similar issues arise in developing a politics over new reproductive technologies; indeed, because these also raise other considerations, the limitations of a politics based on 'reproductive rights' alone become clearer.

In particular, we have to recognise that increasing the range of choices does not always lead to greater real freedom, for some 'choices' may be more available than others and the introduction of a new possibility may affect the range of alternatives on offer. For example, it may be that prior to the public acceptance and availability of abortion in Britain, a young woman finding herself pregnant would have had more moral claim on the father of her child for emotional and material support than she does today for a child she has 'chosen' to bear by refusing to have an abortion.

Of course, it can be said that the choice that is less available to her today, that of greater dependence on a man, is one that she 'ought not' in some sense to want to choose anyway; but we must recognise that many young women do make such choices today and, given the lack of opportunities for women in our society, may indeed be sensible to do so on material grounds if no other. One can hardly expect women who are involuntarily pregnant to be more likely than others to reject the main form of 'security' our society offers to women. The reason, in this example, why the freedom to choose one option closed off another was that the ability to call on the option of marriage depended on the woman's weakness and her lack of alternatives. But women in our society do live under such constraints in which a legal weakness may be to their advantage in exerting moral persuasion; therefore, the extension of some freedoms may in fact curtail others.

Similar problems could arise with prenatal diagnosis. A pregnant woman may choose to have her fetus tested in order to be able to make the choice as to whether to prepare herself for bearing and raising a handicapped child or to have an abortion. But the availability of such tests and the knowledge they provide may in practice constrain rather than broaden her choices. If prenatal diagnosis followed by selective abortion becomes general practice, a woman who chooses to bear a child with a predictable disability may find that currently available welfare services become even more restricted and that, having made her 'own' decision to bear a handicapped child, she is expected to cope on her own too. Such women are already being talked of as 'selfish', and selective abortion following prenatal diagnosis is supported not only by almost the entire medical profession but also by many politicians who are otherwise anti-abortion.

Prenatal testing can also be used to allow the sex of a child to be 'chosen'. Already in India, some private clinics offer amniocentesis, nominally to detect Down's syndrome, where the real aim is to discover the sex of the fetus. Given the value such a society puts on sons and the heavy economic burden that the need to provide dowries for daughters places on a family, it is a safe assumption that the fetuses that have been aborted as a result of such tests are female[6]. But whose choice would that have been? Some women may have been pressured into abortions by husbands or their families, and such late abortions are painful and inevitably distressing procedures. Others may have made the 'choice' themselves because they themselves wanted to bear a son and have felt no direct pressure from others, but it would be difficult to call such a choice 'free' when it results from the low value put on women. Doctors in some parts of Britain have been advised not to tell women the sex of their fetus. Could this form of medical paternalism in practice be a protection for the woman? Or would women be better off for the availability of that particular choice?

What then does the 'right to choose' mean for women, living as we do in an unequal society? If we question whether the right to choose has been genuinely exercised when a woman chooses to abort a female fetus because of the greater value put on sons, should we not also do so when she aborts a fetus with Down's syndrome because society does not provide sufficient support to make raising a mentally handicapped child a choice she can contemplate? And what about the woman who chooses an abortion because her low woman's wage does not make single parenthood, even with a healthy child, economically feasible? Have any of these women really exercised a right to choose?

Reproductive decisions, like all others, are always made within a material and cultural context. To see the context providing the options, and the individual making the choice, is only one way to look at such a situation: the one favoured by the ideology of an individualistic society. The responsibility for the outcome can then be placed on the individual who made the choice, rather than the social conditions under which the 'choice' was made. An alternative way to look at the situation would be to see the context as constraining, ruling out what might otherwise be alternative courses of action, even at times to the point of effective determination.

One study found that women facing the decision whether to abort or bear a fetus they knew would be handicapped often talked about the decision they made, whichever way it went, as their 'only choice'[7]. This contradictory phrase sums up neatly the problem with the notion of freedom of choice in situations where one action is undertaken only to avoid even more dreadful alternatives. The emphasis such women would put is on the lack, not the availability, of choice that the combination of their social and medical conditions imposes on them.

In normal speech, the notion that we have of 'free choice' does not encompass all situations in which choices are made. For example, we do not talk about a prisoner offered the choice between drug treatment or continued imprisonment as having freely chosen the drug treatment. Few women make their reproductive choices in situations in which their physical, material and emotional circumstances are ideal. Such circumstances may well cause a woman to make a different choice than she would have if circumstances had been different. If she would have had the child had she been able to afford it, had better support for the disabled been provided or had more value been put on daughters, then it is circumstances rather than the woman who has 'chosen' and free choice is an illusion.

Another problem with the 'right to choose' is that the choices made by individuals may have social effects that are undesirable. Not only are individuals' choices always made within an economic, cultural and political context, but that context is itself affected by the decisions of individuals. For example, the availability and use of prenatal diagnosis may, we have suggested, lead cost-cutting governments, eager to shift the burden of welfare expenditure onto individual families, to claim that parents who could have chosen not to bear a disabled child have to bear the consequences themselves. And we may find that resources for the treatment of disability, instead of becoming more abundant because fewer babies needing treatment are born, are cut on the grounds that women have the right to choose not to bear such a child, shifting the responsibility for their care from the state to their parents. Such actions would make a mockery of the view of prenatal testing as a type of preventive medicine. The willingness of some Conservative MPs, who are otherwise anti-abortion and against state spending, to spend money on the genetic screening of pregnancies suggests that their real motive must be cost-cutting, and that ultimately the funds for programmes to screen for genetic diseases will be at the expense of research and treatment for the effects of such diseases themselves[8].

And this may affect the way disability in general is treated by society. Even if all congenital defects were detectable before birth, accidents and diseases would continue to leave some people with disabilities. An attitude that the disabled should be eliminated, rather than helped with their disability, might leave those who slipped through the net even more subject to discrimination by society. And the major costs would no doubt fall on unrecognised and unpaid women again, who have always been the ones to care for others with disabilities. Women have traditionally taken on this work, looking after members of their family with disabilities, irrespective of whether the disabilities were the result of congenital defects, postnatal disease or subsequent accidents, and without any consideration of individual responsibility for their cause.

Sex selection provides another example of the way that the extension of choice may have results which are socially potentially undesirable. If parents were able to choose the sex of their children what would be the effects on society as a whole? Many studies have shown that in most societies, there is some preference for sons over daughters, more marked in some societies than in others[9]. In China, the one-child policy has led, in some areas, to a greater imbalance in the ratio of boys to girls born than could be naturally expected, suggesting that late abortion of female fetuses or, more likely, female infanticide, may be being practised to ensure that the only child of the family is male[10]. Amniocentesis is currently too expensive a technique to become so widely used as to affect significantly the overall balance of the sexes, but cheaper techniques are likely to become available in the not too distant future.

Even if the prediction that a preference for males will

destroy itself in a relatively short time by making daughters more desirable is correct, there are other effects to consider of parents being able to choose the sex of their children. Might social prejudices against women become further reinforced if parents had a free choice of the sex of their children and chose thereby the most popular combination of a boy followed by a girl – giving the boy thereby not only the advantages of his gender but also those of being the first-born?[11] And what about the dangers of increased gender stereotyping if children were not only raised but created to conform to a particular gender?[12] All these questions raise in a particular apposite way for feminism the way individual decisions about reproduction could impinge on society as a whole.

Choice, Spontaneity and the Limits of Rationality

But leaving aside the effects of the decisions made on society as a whole there are other more personal issues about the making of reproductive choices to consider. It may seem contradictory to argue that the extension of choice, particularly in an area of such personal importance as reproduction, could be anything but a good thing. Being able to make choices about our lives, free from unnecessary interference, is considered in this society to be the very essence of liberty. But even where women have the personal and social freedom to make their own reproductive decisions, choice itself may not in practice always be welcome.

Wherever they give women the chance to make a choice, however limited, new reproductive technologies inevitably also take the spontaneity out of reproduction. What do women feel about a pregnancy that is achieved through the careful planning and time-tabling that in vitro fertilisation (IVF) and prenatal diagnosis involves? Is it qualitatively different from one in which a woman does not deliberately set out to get pregnant, considers pregnancy and childbirth to be largely a matter of chance and accepts that she will eventually have to care for her baby whatever problems arise? Does it change the feelings women have about pregnancy and birth itself if they know they will be having prenatal tests that might lead to an abortion? What do women feel about having to go through a stage, as one writer puts it, of 'tentative pregnancy'; the woman knows she is pregnant but does not yet know if she is going to have a baby?[13]

It is not so much the new reproductive technologies as contraception and abortion that have changed the role of chance in reproduction and introduced the possibility of planned choice. The very term 'family planning' suggests that rationality can be applied within a traditional social institution. And given what we now know about the methods women have used to control their fertility in the past, it may be a myth to think that reproduction has ever been 'free' of planned decision-making. But despite this, even today, some women feel they could only ever make the monumental choice to have a baby as a result of an accident. They may regret the passing of the time when a woman could leave her fate to chance and dislike having to bear that responsibility themselves. For some people, making decisions is never easy and making such important decisions, about whether to bring a new life into existence and in so doing radically change their own, nearly impossible. If we recognise those feelings as worthy of respect, then undoubtedly the existence of reproductive choice is double-edged for such women, for choice once made available cannot then be ignored. As Barbara Katz Rothman has pointed out about prenatal testing: 'In gaining the choice to control the quality of our children, we may rapidly lose the choice not to control the quality, the choice of simply accepting them as they are.'[14] The 'right to choose' may then have become a burden as well as a source of liberation; losing the right to leave things to chance may be the price of gaining the right to make a choice.

It is unlikely that many women entering IVF programmes feel that way. They after all have been badly served by chance and have actively made the choice to do something about it. Nevertheless, a similar question does apply. Some feminist critics of new reproductive technologies fear, in a society which values women primarily as mothers, that infertile women will be willing to take grave risks with their own physical and mental health in order to be given a chance to bear a child. The effects on women's health of the application of reproductive technologies is rarely discussed; yet the operation to remove eggs for IVF can cause appreciable discomfort and risk, and a late abortion carried out after an adverse prenatal diagnosis is a potentially dangerous and extremely painful procedure. Similarly, the low rates of success of IVF and the disappointment most women who attempt it have to face can cause great emotional stress. Because these aspects are rarely talked about, women may discount their importance in choosing to use new technologies. Might some infertile women not ultimately be happier if no treatment were available and, instead of spending weeks, months or years of anxiety about whether it would ever work, had to come to terms with their infertility, freeing themselves to plan a life in which some other worthwhile activity took the place of child-bearing?

This question is raised in a much more acute form about prenatal diagnosis because what is offered to the woman is not just treatment whose outcome is unknown, but the opportunity to make a choice in a situation in which choice is very painful. Nearly all women who choose to undergo amniocentesis do so in order to give themselves the opportunity of choosing whether to terminate a wanted pregnancy. The choice, as indeed is often the case over abortion, is not one that she would ever have chosen to be in a position to make; she can only 'choose' the lesser of two unacceptable outcomes. Is she really better off for being able to choose, and therefore be considered by others and often even herself to carry the responsibility for whatever decision she makes? Choice within liberal ideology implies responsibility too. Responsible individuals are accorded the right of decision-making because they can be expected to bear the consequences of their own decisions. But women all too often have to bear the responsibility without the choice. Unquestionably this is the case when a woman is denied an abortion, but it is also true in a less clear-cut sense when no option is desirable and the element of choice is so much less important than the problems involved in either course of action.

Reproduction is not the only area in which people have to make difficult decisions they might prefer not to make, but in general we do not see planning and decision-making in other areas as something to be deplored or escaped. But around reproduction women can be made to feel guilty for the very act of having chosen, quite apart from the particular choice made. Over the years, women have been successively castigated for choosing to use contraception, abortion and now prenatal diagnosis. An interesting example of this refusal to allow for planned choice arose recently when the British Medical Association recommended that aborted fetal tissue be allowed to be used in brain grafts, to develop cures for such debilitating conditions as Parkinson's disease. They ruled out, however, the use of fetuses *deliberately* conceived for this purpose. Implicitly, therefore, it was the making of the *decision* to create a fetus for this purpose that was considered unacceptable, for the use of a fetus conceived by accident caused no problems. On similar lines, there has been intense debate, even among those who in general support the use of embryos in research, as to whether it is ethical to use embryos which have been created expressly for that purpose or only ones which were originally created for other purposes but happen to be superfluous to requirements. Of course, in both cases there are grounds on which one might wish to protect women from pressure being put on them to conceive a fetus or donate eggs for such purposes. But in neither case does this seem to be what was at issue. Rather it was the use of planned decision-making that seemed to make processes that were otherwise acceptable into ones that were morally questionable. We have to think what it is about reproduction that makes 'rational' decision-making within it feel so inappropriate.

The dominant liberal idea of 'rationality' turns on the pursuit of self-interest. It advocates that in the public world people should be free to make their own decisions, within certain rules laid down by society, based on their own perception of their self-interest. But behind that notion of public life, is a contrasting conception of a domain of personal relations in the home, where people are supposed to behave quite differently; we are all assumed to do what we do for other members of our family because we care about their welfare rather than as a result of self-interest. In particular, mothers are supposed naturally to love their children in a way that is uniquely selfless. This combination of feelings attributed to nature and selflessness is invoked as the very antithesis of 'economic man' (sic) whose self-seeking decision-making in society serves as the model of rationality in public life. In contrast, therefore, rationality and calculated decision-making appear inappropriate to the relations between parents and children, in particular to a mother's love for her children. Given this, the application of rationality must be even more inappropriate to fundamental questions about the existence of children themselves. Children, by this argument, should be conceived and born in love, not produced like commodities, with a continual search for better methods of production to fashion the perfect product.

Feminists should be wary of these arguments for two reasons. First, the introduction of conscious decision-making into the area of reproduction has been, as far as abortion and contraception are concerned, one of the most important steps towards our liberation, towards our ability to lead lives which are fulfilling in themselves, not just through our children. If we are enabled to make further decisions about our reproductive lives, we do not have to adopt the distorted individualistic criteria of the market-place; we do not have to be 'rational', if rational is to be defined so narrowly. But we should also be wary of rejecting rational choice in reproduction for another reason. The contrast between rationality and love is based on a separation between public and private that has limited women's horizons to the domestic arena. And, as we shall see below, the privatising of reproduction to the domestic unit has meant in practice the allocation of responsibility for it to women alone. If women have that responsibility anyway, it is perhaps an illusion to think that we bear it any the less in reality if we are not able to make choices about it.

The Public and the Private

Behind the question of whether rational choice is appropriate to reproductive decision-making lies a view, shared by many political ideologies, of reproduction as a private concern of individuals and their families, more a matter of feeling than thinking, in which the state has no right to interfere. Within this view, reproductive technologies, by bringing doctors, lawyers and administrators into the reproductive process, can be seen to be destroying the privacy of what *should* be a private matter. This view arises partly from a probably rather healthy distaste for the way medicine, technology and the state have been seen to take control in other areas of our lives, but it takes on particular force when applied to 'interference' in reproduction which is seen as a particularly private area in our society.

Feminist historians have shown how the idea of the home as a private haven, separate and run by different rules from the public world of business, government and work, is a product of specific social developments.[15] It was the Industrial Revolution, the consolidation of capitalism as the dominant system of production in England, which turned the majority of the male population – as well as many women and children – into wage-workers. Before this, production by both sexes typically took place within the household, but the new factory employees worked outside their home, which in turn became the place to which they retreated away from the rigours of the public world. Such ideas about the home have never been a reality for women, because women have always had work to do at home, whether or not they also had a job. Yet the *idea* of it has been very powerful, shaping our notions of the 'private' and, in particular, the belief that it is from self-expression in our 'personal' lives that we should gain the most satisfaction.

But the division of life into public and private arenas has a much longer history. Indeed Mary O'Brien argues that it dates from the discovery of the male role in reproduction[16]. Since that time, the desire to acquire a continuity similar to that women have through the power to bear children has led men to build forms of public life that would outlast them and to confine women to a private arena. Whether or not her theory is correct, it is certainly true that the notions of the home and privacy that are dominant in society today are closely tied up with their being the appropriate places for reproduction. So it is not so much a matter of whether or not reproduction is or should remain a private matter, but rather that the very conception that we have of privacy is one developed from the way our society carries out reproduction.

Feminists have been critical of the way the division of activities into public and private spheres tends to devalue the latter and with it the work of women. The notion of reproduction as a private matter is therefore one that feminists should question and have done so in campaigns for public provision of childcare, maternity benefits, healthcare and so on. But while campaigning for public *responsibility* for reproduction, feminists have also rejected the idea of public interference in our private lives and have claimed that women must have the sole right to make their own reproductive decisions.

Traditionalists also argue against interference by the state in private life, but the notion of the bounds of privacy involved is quite different. For them, it is the family that is to be kept safe from outside interference; even though this can mean allowing immense interference in the liberty of individual members of families. For example, the failure of law enforcement agencies to provide women and children with adequate protection from violent husbands and fathers is frequently excused on the grounds that any effective preventative action would interfere with the privacy of family life. But from a feminist point of view, to leave the family as an island free from outside interference is to leave oppressive relations within the family unchallenged. Thus it is important that feminists, who have after all always been critical of the modern nuclear family, do not confuse their support for a notion of women taking control of their own reproductive lives with the right-wing notion of getting the state off the backs of the family; the latter is simply a recipe for the further intensification of male control within the family. Relations within the family, between parents and children as well as between husbands and wives, can be as oppressive to individuals as state interference in our private lives.

The difference between the traditionalist and the feminist positions was well illustrated by Victoria Gillick's campaign to prevent girls under sixteen being given contraceptive advice without their parents' consent. For traditionalists, this was a campaign to prevent 'society', mainly in the form of doctors employed by the state, intervening in the right of parents to control their children's sexuality. Feminist opposition centred on the rights of the girls themselves to define their own sexuality, free from restrictions imposed either by the state or the family.

New reproductive technologies have developed in a political climate in which the Right, particularly in the United States, articulating concern about the 'breakdown of the family', has portrayed feminism as one of its main enemies. The notion that the family or even marriage, is any less important an institution than it has been in the past is certainly questionable; although more families break up, most parents re-marry and most children spend most of their childhood within a two-'parent' family. Nevertheless, certain features of the family have changed dramatically over the past twenty years or so in most advanced western nations. The prevalence of divorce and remarriage has meant that many children are being brought up in households in which one of their biological parents is missing, in some of which another adult is present, who, while not a biological parent, may be fulfilling more of the traditional parental role than the child's 'real' father or, less frequently, mother. Thus, the 'breakdown' of the family has demonstrated that social and biological parenting roles can be split[17].

This is something that is very worrying to conservative thought for whom the traditional family remains the fundamental unit of society. If ties between family members can be shown not to depend on any genetic connection and the family relatively easily reconstituted around other ties, then it becomes apparent that nature cannot be relied upon to preserve either the family itself or the social system which depends on it. And if the family is weakened, what then is left of a social order which is based on the allocation of people, and with them responsibility for their private griefs, to individual families? Who then must carry the can?

For feminists, however, such trends are not necessarily to be deplored. Directly, it may mean that more women are able to escape from unhappy marriages – most of the increase in the divorce rate since the liberalisation of divorce law in 1969 was in divorces initiated by wives[18] – though most single parents, meaning nearly always single mothers, live in far worse economic circumstances than the married or the childless. But the indirect effects of current trends may be more important, showing that neither the family nor parenthood is a biological given and that the strength of most children's ties to their mother rests more on the care received than the biological circumstances in which they were born. In so far as feminism has always stressed that childcare is real work rather than just the blind following of a biological instinct, the demonstration that biological and social parenting can be split can only be welcomed.

New reproductive technologies may also allow a split between biological and social parenting; through sperm, egg or embryo donation, men or women may raise children who are not their genetic offspring. This possibility has raised a wealth of speculation as to who the 'real' parents would be in such cases. But such a question and the anxieties it expresses originate in the social changes outlined above which will continue to be a much larger source of split parental roles than the small number of cases of infertility to which donation might be a solution.

More worrying for feminists is that these same anxieties may have promoted an emphasis on genetic over social parenting, devaluing thereby a woman's role in bearing and caring for children and reducing her contribution to that of the father's. This would be one interpretation of the demand for technological remedies for infertility – to provide a couple with children to whom they have a genetic, not 'just' a social, connection; otherwise, adoption would do. It is difficult to know the extent to which this idea is important to individual parents – studies have shown that some people who seek infertility treatment would not consider adoption, but many are following both routes, and the development of new reproductive technologies has coincided with the decline in the availability of babies for adoption[19].

Nevertheless, that the most desirable baby is one's 'own' is undoubtedly a popular view and lies behind much of the reporting of the successes of new reproductive technologies. Attitudes are in general much more favourable towards those technologies that provide a couple with children who are their own genetic offspring, than to those where any separation of the roles of biological and social parents results. And it is surrogacy, where a woman bears a child with the explicit aim of giving it away – a further splitting of the maternal role – that has received the widest condemnation.

The traditional family, with its specific form of relation of parents to 'their' children, is a fundamental unit of our society – that is why traditionalists are keen not to see it shaken. But that same family also produces relations between husbands and wives and between parents and children that are oppressive to both women and children. New reproductive technologies may help more couples to become proper families, while at the same time challenging the views upon which the idea of the traditional family rests.

Access to Reproductive Technologies

Legal rights to reproductive choice do not guarantee women access to the means to make those choices a reality; this is well known for abortion, where women have been denied abortions by poverty, prejudice and other unfairnesses in the face of apparent legal opportunities. With the reproductive technologies we have been discussing, which are much more expensive and where a relatively small number of doctors have the power to give or withhold treatment, the gap between legal rights and actual availability is potentially much greater. Our discussion so far has talked about the choice to use reproductive technologies as though they were a reality for everyone, as though all women had access to high-tech forms of infertility treatment and prenatal diagnosis. But currently, and in the foreseeable future, the situation is far from that. Talk about new reproductive technologies today and you are talking about a highly expensive elitist form of medicine, akin to transplant surgery, which costs too much to be available to more than a tiny proportion of the women who might conceivably wish to make use of it. For this reason, some people feel that debates about the ethical and political fine details of new reproductive technologies are just a waste of time. Instead, they would argue, such technological fixes should be seen for what they are, primarily toys for the rich, which on class grounds feminists concerned about the real conditions of the mass of women should have no truck with.

This is particularly true of IVF and the other high-tech forms of infertility treatment. The costs per treatment are extremely high with a very low success rate[20]. This has led to the argument that the money spent on such treatments should instead be directed to preventive healthcare, earlier detection of gynaecological infections for example, that might prevent the cause of infertility in the first place. We do not know of any research which has worked out how effective a preventive programme of the same cost as current expenditure on infertility treatment would be, but it certainly looks likely that, for the same money, far more women could be prevented from becoming infertile than could be helped to bear children through IVF or other high-tech means. If infertility is something that society should be concerned with, then on a societal level that would be money better spent.

But some critics would go further and claim that the treatment of infertility is anyway not a worthwhile societal aim, when, on a world scale, the problem is too many, not too few, babies[21]. But against this it can be argued that it is not the existence of too many people that constitutes the 'population problem', rather it is the way the production and distribution of resources are organised which results in poverty for so much of the world's population. Further, it is a mistake to think that it is any easier to limit the number of children women have than to alter the distribution of resources. So far direct attempts to limit population growth have been remarkably unsuccessful in nearly all cases. The main exception to this has been in China, where a population programme did for a period have some success, but this case can be used to support the argument for social change as being the first step[22]. For China's population programme was but one stage, and not the first stage, of a revolutionary transformation of that society. In general it seems, population programmes can hope to work only if they change the conditions under which men and women see their need for children. Thus, measures to reduce the insecurity which traditionally is coped with by having a large family, improving the status of women and reducing childhood mortality so that fewer children need to be born to provide for their parents' old age would be more effective ways of alleviating poverty than population programmes aimed at persuading or coercing women into having fewer children.

By this argument then there is nothing inherently good or

bad about having children, and if money is to be spent on giving women reproductive freedom at all, it is just as well spent on preventing or coping with infertility as it is on providing the means for women to have fewer children. Feminists have been careful to distinguish the grounds for their support for contraception and abortion provision, to give women the power to determine when, if and how often they bear children, from those of the population controllers who want women to bear fewer children. If population control does turn out to be necessary it can be achieved most effectively and humanely by changing the conditions in which people make their reproductive decisions, not by limiting their ability to make those decisions or even denying them the opportunity of making them at all.

In providing for fertility control and infertility treatment, there is of course a conflict between resources spent in one way and resources spent in another, but these are not absolute conflicts between two things which would undermine each other; both are aspects of giving women control over their reproductive lives. And there remains, of course, the overall question of resources: the difficulty of balancing resources spent on enabling women to have reproductive choice with other worthwhile social goals. Within such a balance, feminists may be more likely than others to put some of their money on reproductive freedom. But if we wish to spend this money as effectively as possible, this will be on preventive care, putting high-tech treatments on our agenda as a luxury to be afforded only when the best preventive programme has been set up.

But this plan of how we might like to see resources used, which is certainly worth campaigning for, ignores the way medical treatment such as IVF is actually funded at the moment. Feminists, like the other interested pressure groups, do not have the power to transfer the enormous resources currently spent on high-tech medicine to other more effective, preventive programmes. In this context, do we wish to ban the expensive technological treatments, do we wish to restrict them to those who can pay for them themselves or do we wish to argue for their provision by the National Health Service out of public resources, and if so at what level?

The argument for banning expensive techniques is that it would put an end to the illusions they foster: their existence may give all women false hope and mistakenly encourage them to continue trying their reproductive luck, when the chances for the vast majority of women are so low, both of ever getting onto an IVF programme and of then succeeding in having a baby. Further, if those illusions were removed, then perhaps women would value the preservation of their own fertility more highly, and take fewer risks with it – of infection, for example – realising how small the chances of doctors being able to do anything about infertility were. It might also cause women to put pressure on governments to fund preventive programmes. However, such a strategy raises the question whether the interference with the reproductive freedom of women who would choose to use such techniques is justified for such hypothetical gains.

The 'libertarian' answer is to let those who want to spend their own money use the techniques, but not to spend public resources on them. This means that only the wealthy will have access to them, a situation which compounds the unfairness of current economic inequalities. It does, however, leave policy-makers with maximum resources to spend on preventive healthcare or any other worthwhile goals, yet at the same ensuring that the research which lies behind IVF, and may have other more generally useful spin-offs, will continue to some extent.

The third alternative is to put some public resources into providing IVF for those women who cannot afford to pay for it themselves. This, the current solution in Britain, is fraught with problems. Unless those resources are very large, they will help only a small proportion of the women who could benefit from IVF. Even if the resources were sufficient to treat everyone, only a small proportion of those treated would succeed in having babies, so an element of unfairness would still be there. The existence of IVF programmes on the National Health Service (NHS) may produce an unwarranted degree of complacency among some doctors – believing that their profession can now do something about infertility – which they may transmit to women, when in practice very few women can be helped.

That not all women who might be able to benefit from IVF can be treated on current resources produces a rationing problem. Doctors select those they will treat. For private sector doctors this means choosing from a relatively small pool, selected by their ability to pay, and some private doctors may be able and willing to treat everyone who comes to them. But on the NHS, waiting lists may get so long that some selection among those on the waiting list *has* to be made, otherwise age alone will become the criterion, and only women who register young enough will receive treatment before they are too old to be medically acceptable.

Doctors forced to choose in such circumstances cannot but allow their own prejudices to determine which women are to receive treatment. Those whose lifestyles fall outside conventional norms, such as single women or lesbians, may be seen as less worthy of treatment, particularly when doctors feel themselves bound to consider the interests of others beyond their own patients, in particular, those of any child that might be born as a result of treatment. IVF specialists tend to see themselves as having a much more direct role in bringing a particular child to life, and therefore having more right to judge whether this is a good thing, than doctors involved in the sort of infertility treatment that would enable a woman to have a child by more conventional methods. Media accounts of technological successes in the reproductive field back up this view of the doctor's responsibility; they are often accompanied by a picture of the mother, medical specialist and 'their' baby. For reasons like these, feminists have, in general, tended to favour 'low-tech' forms of healthcare, in which self-reliance and personal responsibility for one's own health are stressed, rather than those which allow members of a paternalistic medical profession to take control and access to be limited by prejudice, financial resources or legal controls.

Prenatal diagnosis also raises issues of resources, though perhaps less serious ones. Currently in Britain, women over a certain age (this varies from one health authority to another), and women known to be at risk of bearing a child with a genetic disease, will be offered amniocentesis on the National Health Service. Those with a lower risk can have the test privately. From the point of view of overall resources this makes sense if the aim is to *prevent* the birth of such children; by choosing the group of women most at risk, the costs of the test are going to be outweighed by the savings to the health service from having to provide for a reduced number of handicapped children later. For women of lower risk the costs of the test may not be outweighed by resulting savings.

But from the point of view of the individual this may seem very unfair; they may still not wish to bear a handicapped child and want the reassurance the test can provide. For them the considerations of costs to the National Health Service may be a very hard-hearted way to look at it. Indeed, if the aim of the health service is to relieve suffering it could well be argued that the test should be made available to more women than would be justified on cost-benefit grounds alone.

The other danger of this concentration on prenatal diagnosis as a method of saving money is that it takes the woman's choice as a result of the test for granted. Many doctors require a woman to agree to the termination of an affected pregnancy before giving her an amniocentesis[23]. But women have other motives for wanting prenatal diagnosis. Even women who would never consider an abortion might like to prepare themselves for the birth of a handicapped child. And probably most women would like the, albeit partial, reassurance about the health of their fetus that prenatal testing provides, even if many are not prepared to take the risks involved in current methods of testing.

Prenatal diagnosis, however, also raises another problem about access to reproductive technology. It is not only single women, lesbians and black women who find access to the benefits of reproductive technology particularly difficult. Possibly the group whose right to make their own reproductive choices is least respected are women with disabilities. Whether or not they should bear a child is often seen almost entirely in terms of their disability. If a woman has a disability that can be inherited, then she is likely to be heavily dissuaded from having a child and access to help with infertility almost certainly denied. On the other hand, in so far as she agrees with that view of her disability, then prenatal diagnosis may enable her to have a child that she would not have risked before. The existence of prenatal diagnosis can thus be double-edged for women with disabilities and those who know themselves to be carriers of a genetic disease. On the one hand the possibility of diagnosis may intensify attempts to limit their reproductive freedom, on the other hand it may give some of them their only real chance to exercise reproductive choice.

In this chapter, we have questioned in a number of ways whether 'A Woman's Right to Choose' is an adequate principle to guarantee reproductive freedom to women in our society. The issues immediately become more complicated when that freedom is extended to cover situations in which women choose to have a wanted child, rather than those in which they demand the right not to have an unwanted child. We have considered whether the pressure to become a mother in our society leaves women genuinely free to refuse, or choose, motherhood, whether choice in such situations is always desirable and whether rational decision-making should be considered appropriate to our reproductive lives. We have also looked at where anxieties about reproductive technologies seem to come from, uncovering their cause in numerically much more significant changes in society. And finally, we considered whether reproductive technologies really increase choice for women, since they are available to so few women and the conditions under which they are offered may be unacceptable to many.

This chapter has examined some of the societal issues raised by reproductive technologies and what they appear to offer women. However, our discussion so far has not focused on the scientific and technological processes that give rise to such technologies in our society. This is another theme in the public discussion of reproductive technologies and raises a number of questions about the way feminists have seen science and technology, which are explored in the next chapter.

2. Science, Technology and Nature: Women's Friends or Foes?

The 'new reproductive technologies' cropped up in novels long before any of them became a reality. Indeed, the term 'test-tube baby', inaccurately applied to modern technology, comes from a novel by Aldous Huxley. His *Brave New World* depicts a future society in which babies, genetically programmed to have socially required characteristics, are artificially produced in test-tubes. Huxley's vision was of a dystopia, a society from which we were expected to recoil in horror, and his novel is often cited as a warning of the danger of reproductive technology.

Some feminist writing has had a more benign view of artificial reproduction. In *Woman on the Edge of Time*, Marge Piercy depicts a utopia in which babies are produced artificially in order that women and men can form equal attachments to them; furthermore, technological intervention allows men to breastfeed too, as a result of hormone injections. And in one of the most widely cited texts of the modern women's movement, *The Dialectic of Sex*, Shulamith Firestone sees the development of artificial reproduction as the key to women's liberation. Because 'the end goal of feminist revolution must be . . . not just the elimination of male *privilege* but of the sex distinction itself' the 'reproduction of the species by one sex' has to be replaced by artificial reproduction[1]. Implicit in her approach was a view of science and technology as potentially liberatory, a science that women in the future could seize and use for their own ends. In contrast, the natural state of pregnancy was, to Firestone, 'barbaric'; the 'temporary deformation of the body of the individual for the sake of the species' from which women could be released only by breaking that tie to nature.

The view that woman's inferior position in society is a consequence of biology, and in particular her child-bearing role, has a long history. Traditionalists, as we have seen, think of women as inevitably tied to their biology, so that the project of women's liberation is doomed to failure: women's behaviour and social role are determined by their biological difference from men, and, in particular, they are forever constrained by their 'natural' role in childbirth and lactation.

Religious traditions also tend to appeal to the notion of 'nature', and argue that we shouldn't interfere with it; in Christianity, for example, this takes the specific form of disapproving of interference as 'against God's will'. For the Roman Catholic Church the central problem with most reproductive technologies is the separation of sex and reproduction, for it believes that God allowed (marital) sex only in order that reproduction could occur. It is this belief that led to Catholic objections to any form of contraception that does not involve sexual abstinence. But curiously enough, they also use the argument the other way around; it is also wrong to procreate without any sexual act taking place. Ways of overcoming infertility that do not involve sexual intercourse are equally sinful.

The Catholic Church is unique amongst the major Western religions in having a consistent theology that works against practically any conceivable technological change that might affect reproduction. Other religions tend to be a little less hardline. But they all tend to distrust technological change and interference in what God has ordained as natural reproduction. This is not surprising. Religious ideas, because they invoke an unchanging god – like a static conception of nature – have on the whole tended to oppose change.

Yet it is not only change that is feared; human nature itself is under threat. Leon Kass, a biochemist and doctor who writes extensively about ethics and biology, has, for example, questioned the development of reproductive technologies from a traditionalist standpoint. For him:

> Important practical challenges to individual freedom and dignity arise at every turn, most often as inescapable accompaniments of our ability to do good . . . freedom is challenged by the growing powers that increasingly permit some men [sic] to alter and control the behavior of others, as well as by the coming power to influence the genetic make-up of future generations.[2]

Kass sees reproductive technologies as the lynchpin of a terrible fate that awaits us, the very loss of our humanness. Scientists, caught in the liberal trap of believing that their truths are morally neutral, are, he suggests, carrying us into an unnatural science. Applied to the field of reproduction, this 'unnatural science' is one which, instead of allowing us to marvel at nature, begins to threaten our very existence. His inherently conservative concern with the threat to the social structures of marriage and the family lead him to ask:

> Would the laboratory production of human beings still be *human* procreation? Or would not the practice of making babies in laboratories – even perfect babies – mean a degradation of parenthood? . . . Transfer of procreation to the laboratory will no doubt weaken what is for many people the best remaining justification and support for the existence of marriage and the family.[3]

To counteract this trend, Kass suggests a more 'natural' natural science, presumably one that does not try to interfere with the marvels of reproduction. It would, of course, be one that defends the status quo; women and men within this 'natural' science have predetermined roles. And within it,

> . . . a more profound understanding of 'the body' would refute the unnatural and so-called humanistic claims that intelligence or gender-specific roles . . . have no biological basis and are strictly human or cultural creations.[4]

So what such traditionalists want is a science that is *more* imbued with the values of this society, and which consequently shows more concern for the way in which the knowledge it creates can be used to undermine the traditional structures of society. Science, that is, should be more concerned to defend the status quo than to follow the 'unnatural and humanistic claims' of, among others, feminists. Put like this, of course, feminists could have little sympathy with these aims.

Feminists have, on the contrary, usually rejected the idea that our behaviour is determined by our biological difference from men, and have, in particular, exposed the inadequacies of the idea that women are closer to 'nature', while men are closer to 'culture'. Rather, feminists have emphasised that what is seen as 'natural' or 'cultural' are themselves a product of our society; their meanings constantly change.[5] A corollary of that is that it is also not possible to define 'technology' as something wholly unnatural. Feminists may welcome the diaphragm or various methods of 'natural' birth control, because they enhance women's control over conception, but they are not really more natural. Planning the birth of one's children by using temperature charts is as much an artefact of human culture as, say, contraceptive pills.

Women, indeed, should be particularly wary of attempts to resist change on the basis of it being unnatural. Appeals to the 'natural' differences between the sexes have, after all, been used to keep women in oppressed positions for centuries – women have been told it is unnatural for them to enter higher education, to choose any lifestyle other than heterosexual marriage, to choose not to have children, for example. And traditionalists today, by claiming that 'human nature' is impossible to change, have justified the continuation of all the most oppressive aspects of our current man-made and male-dominated society. The fallacy of such arguments is two-fold: first, the status quo they defend is never in itself a natural one, but one existing in and shaped by society. Beliefs about women and higher education have, for instance, changed considerably in this century. Secondly, in a male-dominated society, that status quo will invariably be one that favours men. Change from such 'natural' states is exactly what feminists should be fighting to achieve.

Moreover, just as there is no 'natural' status for women within our society, there cannot be a more 'natural' science of the kind Kass proposes. In any society, science and technology are not neutral; they are created out of the practices of that society, and inevitably embody its social values. In the patriarchal capitalist societies of the West, the forces that have the power to shape technology are far removed from women's influence or interests; as a result, women's relationship to technology remains firmly within established gender lines.

Whether we consider technological change in processes of production (such as the introduction of new domestic appliances, or new office technologies) or the technologies involved in reproduction, women rarely have much input into planning future technologies. Several feminists writing about technology have emphasised both women's absence from the processes of design and development, and how the products that emerge from those processes embody the values of the society that created them. Women's subordination is, effectively, built into the material as well as the social world.[6]

Although many have questioned the assumption that science is neutral, it has been in the late twentieth century that doubts have been widespread. To many people now, science and technology may indeed provide all kinds of wonders, but some of the products of science also threaten our very existence. Science, as more people now realise, is intimately linked to social and political values: science simply does not proceed only in pursuit of neutral facts. Rather, our lives are threatened by nuclear weapons and biological warfare because governments put a great deal of money into 'defence' research; such research cannot be politically neutral.

Awareness of this 'other face' of science has inevitably led to a marked distrust of science and scientists. Scientists could hardly be unaware of this distrust; some are themselves worried by the uses to which scientific knowledge is put. But this does not necessarily dent their belief that science is neutral. A consistent, and widely held view, is that science itself produces nothing more than facts: it is society that is responsible for the use, or abuse, of that knowledge. So, according to this view, the new reproductive technologies are based on morally neutral facts about human reproductive biology, and the uses to which they are put are, on the whole, benign.

A second, related, assumption widely held about science is that it embodies advance, that it is progressive because it adds to the fund of human knowledge by rational scientific enquiry. Producing technologies is a response to that advance; new technologies constitute progress. The idea of scientific progress has been significant in our culture; from the beginning of the scientific revolution during the Renaissance, Western society has, on the whole, upheld beliefs that science enables humankind to control nature, and that this in turn means progress.

One pitfall of the science-is-progress view is that science and technology seem to be guided inexorably by their own dynamics. This aspect has been described as a form of 'technological determinism'; more generally, this is the belief that technological factors (such as the invention of steam-powered engines, say) in themselves generate social and economic change. One extreme example would be the belief that the invention of the typewriter in and of itself led to secretarial work opening up to women. Science and technology, according to these views, are independent of social forces in their creation, yet they have considerable power to determine the social future. Feminists have repeatedly questioned both these views of science and their implications, emphasising instead that the development of new technologies is profoundly affected by the distribution of social power. So, for example, word-processors have been developed not to make life easier for office workers, but to speed up their work thus enabling employers to save money by employing fewer workers and to exert more control over the work. It is the social context in which a technology is created, rather than the technology itself, which initiates change.

A third assumption underlying research into reproduction is that it is responding to social need; that is, that the technologies have been developed for socially beneficial reasons – to help women to bear the children they desire. In so far as these technologies might be used for less desirable ends, some people believe, that is a problem for society and the state, which should enforce appropriate controls. Robert Winston, one of the more outspoken doctors involved in IVF work, arguing in favour of continued research on embryos, concluded that,

> . . . it is imperative that such work is properly controlled by governments. Nobody wants to see Frankenstein experiments, even were these possible. However, many doctors agree that not to continue with such valuable work would be a disaster[7].

That is, the responsibility for the proper prevention of abuse lies outside science and scientists: it must instead fall to law-makers. Science and scientists in this view escape all blame for the effects of the knowledge they discover or create. This liberal view of science encompasses a fairly benign, somewhat unworldly image of scientists, innocently pursuing the truth or simply responding to 'social need' without heed to the consequences. That the consequences may turn out to be disastrous for humanity should not be blamed on science. Society should, and implicitly can, control its uses. What society should not control – and ultimately would fail to control even if it tried – is the growth of scientific knowledge itself.

One problem with this prescription is the meaning that can be given to 'society'. In practice, reference to 'society' in this context usually means control by the state through, for example, legislation and government guidelines. But the state cannot be separated from industrial and commercial interests; it is these that are, ultimately, the forces governing uses or abuses of science. What reference to 'society' does not tend to mean is any sort of 'democratic' control. As radical critics have often lamented, this leaves most people – the constituents of 'society' – without any power to exert control over science and technology. Women as a group, especially, lack the power to influence it. As a result, it is not only distrust that many women feel about the direction of science in our society: it is also despair and powerlessness.

Feminist Responses to the Science of Reproduction

Recognising that despair, some feminists have examined the social context in which new reproductive technologies are being developed. And they have argued that the reason for the development of at least some reproductive technologies has not been concern for women at all. Rather, there have been more powerful motives behind their development. The first set of motives to consider are those of the medical profession. Within it, gynaecology and obstetrics forms a relatively powerful specialism – not because it has to do with women, but because it is surgical. Gynaecologists reflect the values of the wider society, and tend to view women largely in terms of their potential fertility, so that infertility is seen as one of the most serious medical problems that can befall a woman. Men are not seen simply in terms of their reproductive potential, and there is no equivalent medical speciality to deal with the male reproductive system. So infertility tends to be seen as a woman's problem. Accordingly, there has been much more research on the immediate causes and possible treatments of women's infertility, such as how to deal with blocked tubes, than on anything to do with men's infertility.

There has also been relatively little interest in finding and preventing the underlying causes of infertility, such as the factors which cause women's tubes to become blocked in the first place. In particular, there has been little assessment or research into those instances of women's infertility that are thought to arise from previous medical interventions, such as sterilisation or abdominal surgery, or into the failure by doctors to treat gynaecological infections, such as pelvic inflammatory disease, seriously and fast enough.

However, until recently, medical knowledge of the normal processes of fertilisation and pregnancy was insufficient to enable doctors to do anything much about infertility. With the advent of the new reproductive technologies aimed at alleviating infertility, this has suddenly changed, and with it, the status of the infertility specialist. But even now, not all treatments carry the same prestige; the most prestigious are those that show up the skill of the surgeon and use the newest techniques. Removing eggs and replacing embryos by IVF carry considerably more status than getting involved in the preventive medicine that might have avoided the cause of infertility in the first place.

The second set of forces driving the development of reproductive technologies are the concerns of the large corporations whose market is to be found in modern medicine. Their funding is largely behind, directly or indirectly, the research and development of the new techniques, their backers seeing yet another potential profitable outlet in the drugs and equipment needed by the new treatments for infertility. It is just this involvement that illustrates the inadequacy of the belief that the research is simply responding to 'social need'.

On a smaller scale, the private hospitals and clinics that offer such techniques also operate to make a profit. Even in Britain, less than 10 per cent of current attempts at in vitro fertilisation are provided within the National Health Service, and the role of the private sector in other countries is even larger.

In some cases, medical practitioners themselves have become involved in companies promoting techniques they have pioneered. Perhaps the most famous example of this is the company IVF Australia, set up to sell the expertise of the Monash University IVF team, one of the world leaders, to private clinics throughout the world. One serious objection to the involvement of researchers in business is that it inevitably leads to the direction of research being decided by profitability criteria, and to the temptation for researchers to keep their discoveries secret for commercial reasons. Secrecy not only hinders further progress which depends on the worldwide dissemination of research results, but it also makes any public scrutiny more difficult and works against the interests of patients wishing to be able to make their own well-informed choices about treatment. Much commercial research is, of course, kept secret in precisely this way. But research in reproduction is alleged to be motivated by a concern for people facing infertility. The creation of IVF Australia led one commentator to doubt his previous

> understanding of the representations made by all the protagonists of the technique . . . that the IVF quest sprang from concern, the IVF research was motivated by idealism and the IVF practice was altruistic. Perhaps the more mundane reality now betrayed in the association with 'unidentified business interests' should alert the community to the complications.[8]

Yet there is, some feminists would argue, a still more sinister motive behind the desire of men to get involved in developing reproductive technologies such as IVF. That only women bear children is something men can envy, and has so far ensured a dependence of men on women – if they are to reproduce at all. Now, they argue, men are attempting to remove that last vestige of power from women, to take control of women's reproductive powers too. Ultimately, the argument goes, men could then choose to dispense with women altogether or to use them simply as incubators for embryos artificially conceived and controlled by men. By this argument, current technologies could be but a first step in the eventual extermination or reproductive enslavement of women (for further discussion of this possibility, see Chapter Eight).

Somewhat different questionable motives may lie behind the development of techniques for prenatal diagnosis of genetic defects in fetuses. Raising a child with a degenerative disease can be heartbreaking and many genetic abnormalities lead to disabilities which require a great deal of hard work on the part of the care-giver. Parents, usually mothers, put in most of that work, often with little or no financial support. But there are other costs, too, which fall on the health and welfare services; the extent to which these are borne by the state or by medical insurance varies from country to country. But under almost any system, these are sufficient to make it less expensive to provide prenatal genetic testing and encourage women to abort affected fetuses than to support children subsequently born with severe disabilities. Further problems arise if such an argument is then used to shift the costs further onto the woman herself, on the grounds that she could have chosen to have an abortion.

And again, there is an issue of control here. Several researchers are involved in work in prenatal diagnosis in response to pleas from communities most affected by serious genetic diseases. Nevertheless, as several critics have pointed out, encouraging abortions on grounds of potential genetic handicap could lay the way open for abortions on eugenic grounds, of 'purifying the gene pool'. Just as various forms of contraception are encouraged in developing countries because of a western belief in 'overpopulation' in the third world, so it remains possible that what motivates some researchers is a desire to control who gives birth.

These different motives are not necessarily distinct. Some medical practitioners have indeed made their reputations and a good deal of money out of women's infertility, while some in vitro specialists have displayed particularly chauvinistic attitudes towards women. Doctors who wish to prevent the reproduction of 'imperfect genes' may be motivated primarily by a desire to save money. But this does not mean that researchers are universally driven by such undesirable motives, nor does it rule out the possibility that the new developments may help some women as well.

Technology is a social product, and it is not surprising that such a combination of personal ambition, the profit motive and patriarchal control is evident in technological development: it is certainly not unique to technologies of reproduction. New information technology, for example, has spawned its own brand of machismo in the 'hackers' who devote their lives to computers. And the most successful of their products increase profitability by allowing firms more efficiently to control their workers' ability to labour. Yet information technology has liberatory potential, too, and it would be counterproductive for feminists to reject the use of computers because of dubious motives and social values of their designers. Marge Piercy envisages the use not only of artificial reproduction but also microchip technology in the creation of a more humanitarian and more environmentally conscious society in *Woman on Edge of Time*, and feminists today also campaign for the use of computers to benefit women in our society – to provide more efficient records for cervical screening, for example.

But any liberatory potential of computers does not reside in the technology itself; it also resides in the possibility of women taking control. Similarly, despite claims that domestic appliances help to 'liberate' women from housework, there is nothing instrinsically 'liberating' in these forms of technology; any role they might have in transforming women's domestic labour occurs in a broader context of gender roles.

Still, this is not to argue a simple 'use–abuse' model, where the technology itself is value-free and becomes good or evil only when put to some use. The history of any technological development inevitably affects the form it takes today, and there are undoubtedly some technologies that are so imbued with a particular set of social values that the technology itself seems intrinsically oppressive or liberatory. Chastity belts, for example, seem doomed to an oppressive, rather than liberatory, use: in this case, oppression does seem intrinsic to the product itself, and no amount of 'taking control' could ever change it. All technologies bear the marks of their development in an unequal society, some more obviously than others.

Current developments in reproductive technology are taking place in a society in which women have little power, and in which their bodies are abused. The forms that these technological developments take therefore reflect and incorporate the power and beliefs about women of a largely male medical profession. For example, an advertisement, aimed at doctors, for a new vaginal probe for ultrasound detection of mature eggs, part of the IVF procedure, depicts a group of flying storks carrying babies across the countryside. And there among them is a flying probe, anyway an obvious phallic symbol, carrying a baby too and providing explicit visual representation of gynaecological pretensions, via their technology, to female reproductive powers.

Feminist priorities would, no doubt, have been different in the development of existing technologies; and so our technologies would themselves have been different. But the only ones available to us today, not just in the field of reproduction but in all aspects of our lives, *are* those developed in a capitalist patriarchal society and largely for capitalist/patriarchal motives. Some of these may be used by women for their own benefit – some may not; each new development will have to be considered on its merits. The history of their development by itself does not provide the answer.

Feminists need to be wary of seeing reproductive technologies as *inevitably* leading to a slippery slope towards greater male power. That is to ascribe too much power to the technology itself, a form of technological determinism. Rather, 'It is not technology,' Cynthia Cockburn has pointed out, 'that is out of control, but capitalism *and men*.'[9] The control over women that some writers fear will be intensified by, say, producing babies in the laboratory, does not lie in the technology, but in social organisation – a question of power. Feminists must also beware of the wholesale rejection of science, however critical of it we may be. One strand of feminist critique of science returns to the view of women as somehow closer to nature than men, and questions the idea that scientific knowledge has to be based on abstraction and the taming of nature, methods of thought that it sees as specific to patriarchal societies. Some feminist critics have argued that male science has developed by wiping out earlier female traditions of intuitive, practical, knowledge, more in sympathy with an untamed nature. (Similar arguments have been made about the impact of Western, imperialistic, scientific traditions on the knowledge of nature held by other cultures.) This has, they argue, been particularly true within medicine, with female healers being persecuted as witches in medieval times and their knowledge suppressed. So, their intuitive, holistic understanding of the human body has now been superseded by modern medicine's mechanical view of bodies as little more than the sum of their parts.

But this view is controversial among feminists precisely because it posits women as more 'natural', having virtues that are somehow more in tune with their environment.[10] As we have seen, both the concepts of 'women' and of 'nature' are themselves part of the ideology of a male-dominated society, with their meanings constantly changing. If arguments for a more feminist science are to be based on alleged virtues of women, these virtues must be recognised for what they are – products of women's role in this society. They are not some universal female quality. Such a science might indeed be a better science, but not for being inherently female. Indeed, without recognising that 'natural' can mean different things to different people, it sounds dangerously like Leon Kass' view of a more 'natural' natural science.

Challenging Science

For feminists, a progressive vision of science must be one that challenges, rather than reinforces, the prejudices and constraints of society. Indeed, to the extent that reproductive technology allows us to question the automatic assumption that current social relations of reproduction are inevitable, it can be welcomed. Remembering how much of what appears to be 'natural' is in fact just a product of our society, it is important not to fall into the trap of rejecting challenges to existing practices just *because* they appear to involve going against nature.

Two questions remain for feminist analyses of science and technology. What would a scientific practice that was more acceptable to women be like, and how could it be so transformed? And what attitudes should we have to the practitioners and products of today's science and technology? This book is largely, though not entirely, about the second question. We hope to be able to identify clearly defined issues about new reproductive technologies around which feminism should be able to organise and engage in debate.

In writing this book, we have tried to identify issues that raise specific moral or ethical concerns for feminism, rather than treating reproductive technologies as just a great ragbag of patriarchal tinkering with our bodies. We remain unconvinced that the solution to these concerns is simply to oppose all reproductive technologies, not least because this stance does not clearly identify what feminists should *do* to organise around these issues. To this end, we have tried to separate out those forms of technological intervention that are currently available from those that are still far off, or even simply unachievable. Issues around prenatal diagnosis and subsequent abortion raise questions for feminists now; the prospect of a complete male takeover of producing babies is technologically a distant prospect. If it were possible to do it, the society in which it happens will be different, and choices for political struggles will be on different terrain. We believe that one reason why reproductive technology seems to excite so much opposition is because feminists have yet to identify the sites on which to organise our political struggles. Given the speed at which things change within this field this is an urgent task.

But underlying these questions is a broader one about the practices of science and technology in general, and the way feminists hope to change them. Writings about reproductive technologies often take the practices of scientists as inviolable, as though they could not be challenged by feminists from within or without. It is on this basis that some feminist writing about new reproductive technologies has tended to argue that we should simply refuse them. We believe that to be an unnecessarily pessimistic and possibly dangerous outlook for women, because we can ill afford to ignore struggles about the way science itself is conducted.

For what chance might we have, even if this was what we wanted, to stop the development of such technologies? Just because science and technology are so clearly *not* in women's hands, trying to stop it altogether from the outside is a hopeless quest. We have, therefore, whether we like it or not, to engage in a struggle *with* science and technology, to make them more in tune with women's needs. We have to develop our own 'appropriate technologies' reflecting women's needs (just as agricultural work in the Third World had to develop technology appropriate to local needs and conditions, after the dismal failure of Western high-cost technology). Science today is clearly not directed towards empowering women. But science is not unique in that and a major theme of feminist projects has been to insist that feminism challenges and transforms all aspects of society in which women are at a disadvantage. Why then should we abdicate responsibility for transforming particular types of sciences?

Our principal project, then, is one of examining and analysing the questions posed by current new reproductive technologies: but it has set us a wider agenda, too, to think about how we might struggle around creating a better scientific practice in the future, one that is more responsive to our needs. For that reason, after examining current reproductive technologies and the issues they pose in Part Two, we shall return to consider questions about science and technology in the future. But our focus will be not only on what might, or might not, be about to happen, but also on the forms of resistance women can mount: how, that is, we might affect what that future might be.

3. The Medicalisation of Reproduction: Justifications and Assumptions

In Part Two, we will discuss what goes wrong when people become infertile or suffer from genetic disease, and what the medical profession now know about the underlying biological processes. Here, however, we explore some of the assumptions often used to justify research into reproduction and the further 'medicalisation' of such human experiences: research into potential causes of infertility, for example, is sometimes justified on the grounds that women want medical treatment, or that the treatment aims to correct a disease or disorder, or an 'unnatural' state. In other contexts, appeals to the scientific discoveries about early human development are used either to justify or condemn abortion, in vitro fertilisation (IVF), and research on human embryos and disease. This justification, too, makes many assumptions.

In this chapter, we look at some of the implications for women of the growing influence of medical and scientific thinking centred around reproduction. People have always desired to control the processes of reproduction – but, in practice, it has been left largely to women to effect that control, however sporadically. Feminist historians have pointed to the rise of the predominantly male medical profession over several centuries, and how it has gradually eroded what little control women may have had. In this century, contraception and abortion – once activities that were probably largely in women's hands – are now firmly in doctors' control.

Reproduction has, of course, always taken place in women's bodies, and until this century, doctors understood very little about its mechanisms. Such methods of contraception that existed usually relied on some form of abstention (as required, for example, by the 'safe period'), or on 'barrier' methods (such as the condom) that prevented sperm and egg from meeting. But the end of the nineteenth century saw the birth of a new branch of science called endocrinology (the study of endocrine glands and their secretions, hormones). This led to much greater scientific understanding of reproductive physiology, and hence, to much more *specific* forms of contraception such as the Pill. The contraceptive pill, like many new treatments for infertility, uses analogues of our bodies' hormones and can offer a very fine control over the details of reproduction. But this focuses attention on high-tech solutions rather than on the reasons why the infertility may have arisen or on why it represents such a problem for women.

Current developments aimed at intervening in reproduction echo previous technologies also in the way the profit motive has controlled their supply. Although scientists discovered in the 1940s that certain hormones could block the processes by which eggs are normally released, it was not until the pharmaceutical industry began to produce and promote them in the 1960s that contraceptive pills became widely used. And so it is with techniques such as IVF: however wonderful the skills, expertise and dedication of the medical teams which practise it, it has begun to take off due to the profit-motivated investment by drug companies and the private clinics which provide most of the treatments.

'Women Want It': Research as a Response to Social Need

So developments in science and medicine may potentially increase the control of a largely male medical profession over women's reproduction. Many researchers find such developments unproblematic, however, because they see research and development of reproductive technologies as responding to social need, that 'women want it'. Research into improved methods of contraception, for example, may be justified in terms of global population (particularly in developing countries), that people everywhere want safer, more efficient forms of contraception.

A justification for research into causes of infertility is similarly that women want it; indeed, that infertile women are 'desperate' and will go to considerable lengths to have a baby. The notion that women 'want' it is closely linked to the idea of infertility as a disease or disorder – something that falls within the purview of modern medicine, and which by definition needs 'treatment'. Unlike research into contraception, however, the 'market' for infertility research and treatment is not global; infertility is a problem throughout the world, although it is only in the richer, developed nations that medical treatment on any scale has emerged.

Yet how much of these developments can be attributed to 'consumer demand'? There is no doubt that discovering you are infertile can be traumatic. It can trigger feelings of failure or inadequacy, or a sense of helplessness; for both men and women it can engender identity crises because it seems to strike at the heart of our sense of what it means to be gendered, to be female or male. Naomi Pfeffer and Anne Woollett, in their book *The Experience of Infertility*, quote the reactions of a number of women to the discovery of infertility: one, for example, felt that

> It's such a personal thing, a secret I was harbouring. My body didn't belong to me and I didn't like it. My self-image was badly dented through all of this. I turned in on myself. I felt as though I wasn't a proper woman.[1]

Women experiencing infertility frequently report feelings of isolation and rejection, often from friends and relatives who themselves have children[2]. Some fear rejection from husbands or lovers (a fear that can easily become reality in some societies). Given cultural beliefs about the purpose of marriage, and the importance of reproduction within it, it is no surprise that many people, both women and men, react to their own infertility with a sense of failure. But the consequences of that discovery are worse for women, particularly if they choose to have treatment. In practical terms, infertility treatments usually mean taking frequent blood and urine samples, frequent trips to hospital clinics, internal examinations and, sometimes, sexual intercourse with their partner to order. The emotional costs of discovering you are not fertile are also usually greater for women. In a society in which women are defined primarily in terms of their capacity to reproduce, infertility inevitably raises particular problems for a woman's sense of herself and of her own femininity. As one woman, interviewed in an Australian study, commented:

> In my most depressive state, I felt a total *lack* of femininity. I reverted to a . . . sort of neuter . . . I felt terribly speyed. It was quite loathsome . . . I didn't *really* believe my body was there.[3]

If finding yourself infertile is so traumatic, then it is not surprising that many women do often seek medical advice. Similarly, most women who have already had a child with a serious genetic disease may wish to try and avoid having another. Without prenatal diagnosis, this can only be done by stopping reproducing altogether, while if prenatal diagnosis is available, they can continue to try to have healthy children.

Nor is it surprising that pressure groups, such as FACT (the Fertility Action Campaign for Treatment), campaign for greater availability of infertility treatment, and many charities now campaign for prenatal diagnosis. So, in these senses, there is some basis for the claims that 'women want it'; in Western countries at least, there has been some 'consumer demand'.

Yet any such 'demands' do not necessarily drive the research, but may simply be one response. Other women may not accept it. Throughout the history of medical interventions in women's reproduction, women have rarely been consulted about their needs; indeed, they have often found ways to resist medical technologies. Ann Oakley suggests that

> The question is: why is it that in relation to any reproductive technology the recurrent medical question is *not* 'Why do women want it?' but 'Why *don't* women want it?' . . . whether it is the contraceptive pill, or seeing the foetus on the ultrasound screen, or amniocentesis to detect handicap, or . . . programmes of genetic counselling or . . . artificial modes of fertilisation, many doctors do not seem to understand that what they have to offer are not universally desired goods.[4]

An even more fundamental problem is that 'wanting' implies the ability to make choices, that women participating in IVF programmes have freely chosen to do so because that is what they want. But where does that motivation come from? As Christine Crowe suggests,

> In a situation where women experience personal condemnation and social stigma because of their infertility and in which the social definition of motherhood necessitates a biological relationship, the question must be asked what *real* 'choices' do infertile women have? To participate in an IVF procedure, with its low 'success rate', or to remain without children, with all its negative implications, seems to represent very little choice.[5]

The assumption that research is a response to women's wants also ignores the fact that many women who may want to overcome infertility will be denied access to this procedure. The more technological kinds of infertility treatment, including IVF, are expensive; even in the West, they are open to only a small minority. Ability to pay is vital, although so, too, is who you are. Many women are denied access to IVF programmes because, say, they are lesbian or disabled. And the large numbers of women living in the Third World who are infertile may have no access at all, particularly if they are poor and live far away from cities.

Similar inequalities in access to prenatal diagnosis are also widespread. Women in the British communities most affected by specific diseases may want access to prenatal testing, but they do not always get it. Janet Black and Sophie Laws point out that 'no Asian community in this country has been given full information about thalassaemia, so that young people might know about their risks before marriage and childbearing'[6].

'Natural' Fertility

The 'medicalisation' of human reproduction also fuels the notion that infertility is a 'disease' or a 'disorder' – a discrete state of being, and an 'unnatural' one at that. Fertility is, to judge from what we are taught of reproductive biology, the 'natural' state, and pregnancy something that is easily achieved. Yet infertility can sometimes be an adaptation – a self-protecting response – to environmental stresses. The fertility of women in Holland during the famine of 1944 declined sharply, and the fertility of malnourished women who are breastfeeding infants also drops. Severe mental or physical stress, or very low body weight, can also lower a woman's chance of conceiving.

Moreover, none of us is completely fertile throughout our years of menstruation; ovulation, the release of an egg from the ovaries, does not occur in every single cycle, especially in young women who have just started menstruating, and in women coming up to the menopause. The notion of 'natural' fertility means little even throughout the lifetime of an individual woman.

Infertility, moreover, is no more 'unnatural' than fertility is 'natural'. Compared to other animals, humans have a rather low level of fertility. The average rate of conceptions for human populations is only about 20 per cent for each cycle of ovulation; 'the overpopulation of the world with people,' commented one researcher, 'is due not to their efficient reproduction but to their efficient survival'.[7] We are simply not a 'naturally fertile' species.

Many clinicians now claim that infertility is increasing in the population at large. But others debate this conclusion. It is partly a matter of medical definitions: 'infertility' and 'subfertility' generally means being unable to, or finding it difficult to conceive, whereas 'sterility' refers to those people who lack the ability to have children through a lack of eggs or sperm (perhaps because of some congenital defect) or because of surgical sterilisation.

But it is more than a matter of confusion over medical terms. Part of the problem is the lack of information. It can be difficult to assess the scale of infertility – some people are voluntarily childless, for example, and many do not seek medical help. Whatever the reason, there have been very few statistical surveys.[8] Such information as exists suggests that infertility may be quite common, particularly in some parts of the world.[9] In one recent study carried out in England, the researcher estimated that at least one in six couples 'need specialist help at some time in their lives because of infertility'.[10]

Moreover, the criteria used to define infertility may often be inappropriate. Doctors usually assume a couple to be infertile if they have failed to conceive within one year, and then begin medical diagnoses and treatments. But this time-limit confounds an inability ever to conceive with difficulty in conceiving quickly. Some people may simply take longer than a year to conceive – for all sorts of reasons, including emotional and physical stress. Because of growing awareness that doctors can 'treat' some forms of infertility, there is a danger that they increasingly classify such people as 'infertile'. In previous decades, the people concerned would simply have waited.

The inevitable consequence of a growing medical interest is that infertility is alleged to be on the increase. It is difficult to judge whether this is true; but, because of the predominance of the medical viewpoint, little thought is given to the kinds of environmental factors that might give rise to an increase in infertility – exposure to radiation hazards, or chemical pollutants, for example. Nor is much thought given to infertility caused by previous medical interventions.

Despite the possibility that at least some infertility results from environmental hazards or medical mismanagement, the blame for the alleged increase is sometimes placed firmly at the feet of today's 'liberated women'. Many doctors deplore trends towards having babies later in life, as women struggle to combine motherhood with a career. Doctors urge women not to postpone having children until their 30s because infertility increases with age. Other clinicians have blamed infertility on an alleged increase in sexually transmitted disease. Arguments such as these highlight the issue of social control, which are often implicit in 'medical' explanations. More significantly, by blaming women, they divert attention from any consideration of how some infertility could be prevented.

The Sanctity of the Genes

The growth of the medical and scientific world view has also led to an obsession with 'ethical' debates about the moral status of the embryo or fetus – amazingly, usually to the exclusion of any mention of the mother. This preoccupation in turn leads to a justification for further research on embryos. At the core of this focus is the belief that the genes – the unique hereditary material in all the cells of our bodies – define us as individuals from the moment of conception. Another assumption follows from this: that all that fetuses need to do in order to develop is to follow the inherited instructions in the genes. This assumption, we will argue, deflects attention from the role of either the fetus itself or of the mother in fetal development.

Feminists have typically been suspicious of this neglect of the mother: one feminist article summed it up by casting feminists in opposition to 'fetalists'.[11] The general trend in reproductive medicine at present is towards seeing the fetus as patient, an individual in its own right. However laudable the aim of treating, say, fetal disease prenatally, this trend tends to obscure women's role in the process of reproduction.

The idea that women supply little more than nourishment for the growing embryo is one with a long history in Western thought. And, apart from overemphasising the fetus, it is an idea that has, historically, accorded men more importance than women in the processes of reproduction. Aristotle – philosopher-scientist of Ancient Greece – concluded that, because men were the hotter, and more active sex, their 'seed' formed the embryo. Women, by contrast, were colder and more passive. So, he believed, their role must be that of simply housing the growing embryo.

The idea that men's seed is of paramount importance has come down to us through the ages, and is still extant. It is less obvious in discussion of human reproduction – most of us are well aware that egg and sperm contribute roughly equally – but persists in animal breeding. The racehorse industry, in particular, puts an enormous premium on sires, to the relative neglect of the mare's contribution. (This is partly because it is possible to breed hundreds of offspring from one male, so it is easy to work out if that male is producing good quality offspring. But interest in females is increasing now that eggs/embryos can be retrieved surgically, thus making it possible to breed many offspring from one female.)

'Men's seed' was, for most of recorded history, synonymous with semen: the existence of sperm was known until the invention of the microscope in the seventeenth century. In the same century, William Harvey showed, for the first time, that mammals too produce eggs, and that female eggs were essential for reproduction. Not that discovery of the anatomical details of the female reproductive tract completely changed the primacy of the male; for a start, gynaecological textbooks of the seventeenth and eighteenth centuries portrayed vaginas as inside-out penises. Women's anatomy was still considered very much a receptacle, nearly two thousand years after Aristotle.

The discovery of sperm provoked another debate, and one that is important for understanding the background and assumptions to some of the debates about embryos today. Many seventeenth-century observers of sperm saw in them a miniature person; fanciful imaginations saw the head and tail of a single spermatazoon as equivalent to the head and body of an adult. Because of the similarity, it was called a 'homunculus', or little person: there were even jokes about seeing a homunculus taking off its coat! This in turn led to the notion – following Aristotle – that sperm merely matured into the person, beginning its unfolding within a woman's womb. As these potential, miniature people (sperm) are contained inside the adult man, they reasoned, each man contains within him the seeds of all future generations, like a series of Russian dolls.

To be fair, there were those who opposed this idea; this they did by stressing the primacy of the egg which was also seen to contain the generations. But, by the end of the seventeenth century, it was the theory of male seed that became dominant. That dominance is important to our understanding of some of the debates about reproductive technology. It is, of course, not very surprising to feminists that men feel alienated from reproduction, and might want to feel more in control of it;[12] they are, after all, involved biologically only at the moment of fertilisation. The claim that women provide only the nourishing uterus, while men provide seed that develops into an embryo, has historically provided men with some sense of biological continuity, even if it was less obviously provable than women's.

But the other important point about these ideas is that they portrayed embryonic development as *unfolding*. This notion of unfolding from a preformed shape is known as preformationism and has had a surprisingly persistent influence on the way we think about embryos. Preformationism was the predominant way of thinking about embryonic development during the eighteenth century; but by the end of that century, another idea was beginning to gain credence. This was the idea that, rather than unfolding, the various parts of the embryo differentiated out of material which was, initially, quite unformed. This idea was called epigenesis, meaning the active creation of new shapes and forms, and it emphasised that embryos begin by actively *creating* structures from a simple ball of apparently identical cells.

Most biologists who work today on the study of the embryo do not tend to think of development as merely unfolding. Yet that does not seem to change popular ideas. Concern was expressed in the deliberations of the committee chaired by Dame Mary Warnock that human embryos should not be used for research, even in the first fourteen days (that is, before they would become attached to the uterine wall) because they are *human* embryos. While not explicit, this implies unfolding, rather than a process of development in which both fetus and mother play an active part. What is morally repugnant, this view suggests, is the idea of research on an embryo that contains in miniature a future human life. But in what sense is this cluster of cells human?

It is clearly not yet human in that it has obviously not entered human social life. It is said, rather, to have the potential to become human. But the cluster of cells *cannot progress unless they can implant* – at present, that means implanting into a woman's womb. So, the 'potential' for humanness must reside more in the genes that it has inherited from its parents than in the embryo's absolute reliance on a woman's uterus.

In fact, the early developmental stages – the cells that arise from the fertilised egg – are sometimes described as 'pre-embryos'. They do not have an absolute 'potential' to form a human being; rather this potential changes with their stage of development. Even in nature, most, perhaps two-thirds, of fertilised eggs spontaneously stop developing at an early stage. Many fertilised eggs become blocked when they have divided into four cells, the time when the embryo's own set of genes are switched on, if all goes well. Several other fates can await a pre-embryo. It may become a 'hydatiform mole' – its cells forming just support tissue and no proper embryo at all. Or twins may develop, instead of a single individual. Above all, it has to implant itself into the wall of the uterus. If it does not implant at exactly the right moment, its chances of developing further are nil. An 'embryo' begins to develop about sixteen days after ovulation, but the chances of miscarriage are still high. As the embryo develops into a fetus, some eight weeks after ovulation (or ten weeks after the last menstrual period), its chances of surviving to term gradually increase.

Yet despite this uncertainty, many ethical arguments begin from the assumption that a uniquely individual human life is created with each fertilisation. The question of when life begins has always been a thorny one for theological debate, and it is often seen as central to ethical debates about the morality of IVF or embryo research. 'Pro-life' groups increasingly appeal to 'science' to justify their position. For instance, a leading Catholic geneticist, Jerome Lejeune, claims that modern genetics shows that the moment of fertilisation is the beginning of life: 'The genetic make-up of the new human being is established: not a theoretical or a potential human being, but the very human being we will later call Peter, Paul or Magdalene.' As the genes in the egg and sperm mingle together, the unique genetic complement of an individual is established. Therefore, a fertilised egg is sacred and really a person.[13]

There are several responses to this kind of argument. One can claim, on a technical point, that science itself does not justify Lejeune's conclusions. Researchers at Cambridge have established that an embryo's own complement of genes are not 'expressed', that is, they do not begin their work of making proteins, until the fertilised egg has divided twice to form a four-cell embryo. Before then, its development is guided by molecules laid down by the mother as the egg was formed.

In a more basic way, an appeal to science cannot be used to justify ethical concerns about embryos. For life does not begin at fertilisation – egg and sperm, and all our cells, are alive too. John Biggers of Harvard University in Boston has elegantly elaborated this argument.[14] Most living organisms arise from others of their kind by an 'alternation of generations'. One generation, the dominant one in humans, is made up of cells that have two pairs of each set of chromosomes (known as the 'diploid' phase; humans have twenty-three pairs, each consisting of thousands of genes). This generation alternates with the sexual phase, made up of cells with only one pair of chromosomes (the 'haploid' phase). We tend to be unaware of this full life cycle, with its alternation of haploid and diploid cells, because the haploid phase is much reduced in humans and other vertebrate animals – it exists only in the egg and sperm – and is dependent upon the diploid phase. This is not the case in all living organisms, however; in some plants, the haploid generation has a life apart from the diploid and may indeed be the dominant life form. Liverworts and mosses, for instance, follow this pattern.

The point for us is that life is a continuous process, with no beginning and no end (save that of the extinction of a species). Such a biological context brings home the point that science cannot provide the basis for any value judgements we may put on the relative value of haploid and diploid phases. This biological perspective may make us less prone to regard children as possessions. Even our sex cells are not really 'ours' but a separate generation: they are not even identical to our body cells.

Nonetheless, the ethical debates usually rely on the assumption that life begins at fertilisation; the development of the embryo thereafter then depends on the genes it possesses. This emphasis on genes, the genetic make-up of the fertilised egg, brushes over all the uncertainty in early development – whether it will implant, whether it will abort – and gives a false primacy to genetics, just as many earlier biologists did for sperm. In practice, it is not easy to define what is 'human' about genes. Human genes are made up of DNA, of which only a relatively small amount is actually different from, say, our nearest neighbours (other apes). Perhaps more to the point, even genes cannot produce their 'human potential' on their own: they work in interaction with their environment. For the developing human fetus, that includes the mother's body, and her immediate environment.

Scientists can recreate the biological environment sufficiently well for a newly fertilised egg to begin to divide and grow in laboratory conditions: at present, though, embryos soon stop developing in the laboratory. The human potential exists only in the process of interaction between the changing, developing embryo and its *human* environment – a woman. Somehow, the concern with 'human potential' has focused on the genes to the exclusion of much else.

These assumptions, about when life begins and about fetal 'unfolding' from instructions in the genes, underpin traditionalists' claims that, for example, it is morally wrong to conduct research even on embryos less than fourteen days old. Abortion is morally wrong, they claim, precisely because it involves killing a miniature human.

The supposition that we can describe 'fetal rights' that are morally equivalent to, or even supersede, the rights of the mother is based upon the implicit belief that the fetus is a fully-formed human, almost from the moment of fertilisation. Feminists have to question this assumption, not only in relation to our insistence on a woman's right to choose whether to continue with any pregnancy, but also because it is a rhetoric that diminishes the significance of the mother's role in reproduction. There is no biological foundation for this emphasis: we should recognise it for the ideological device that it is.

These three assumptions – that there is a social need, that infertility is unnatural or a disease, and that embryos/fetuses unfold devoid of any context – flow from an increasing reliance on the 'medicalisation' of reproduction. They also serve to justify further research. In Part Two, we look in detail at the biological processes that 'go wrong' in infertility and genetic disease; the three assumptions we have considered here pervade the medical framework in which most women inevitably experience problems of infertility or disease. And as we shall see, they affect the ways in which women might respond to reproductive technologies.

Part 2

4. What Goes Wrong? Reproductive Technologies and Infertility

The last three chapters dealt with the context and some of the assumptions surrounding research into reproductive technologies. In the next four chapters, we begin to look at these developments in more detail. There are, broadly, two kinds of intervention that might be made: those that aim to overcome problems posed by infertility, and those that aim to prevent the birth of children with inherited diseases.

The first kind of intervention aims to overcome the problems of infertility. Medical options include the techniques involved in IVF; these medical interventions can take various forms. Some, such as hormonal 'fertility drugs', are aimed at 'persuading' a woman's body to produce sufficient eggs to enable fertilisation to occur normally. In other cases, it may be impossible for fertilisation to occur naturally – because a woman has blocked tubes, say. The aim then is to bypass the problem by using IVF, for example.

Any woman's experience of infertility – or fertility – depends upon both social and biological processes, acting together. In the social domain, her experience will be shaped by, for example, her economic situation, or the quality of social support she enjoys. It will also be informed by more pervasive social pressures – the pressure on women to find fulfilment through children, for instance, or the pressure on women to have sons. Both women's experience of fertility/ infertility, and our general understanding of what those terms mean, depend crucially on notions of femininity – what it means to be a woman.

Yet women's experiences depend also on biological processes – ovulating, fertilisation, implantation of an embryo, pregnancy itself. For most women, it is only pregnancy that is consciously experienced as a changing biological process (though some women experience ovulation as slightly painful, and some report that they are intuitively aware that fertilisation has occurred). But for women who are less easily fertile, the biological processes have different meaning; infertility may mean, for example, that a woman experiences some part of her body as having failed, of letting her down. And just because most women will seek help from the medical profession to overcome infertility problems, that meaning is often determined by medical understanding of 'what can go wrong' with our bodies.

In the next three chapters, we have organised our discussion around those biological processes. We have done this because, if we want informed debate among women, it is important for us to know what it is that doctors and scientists are seeking to do, and because it is the *medical* (or biological) context in which many women will directly encounter the different interventions. To do this is not to assume that these are the only solutions. What is offered by doctors is an extremely limited range of options, within a strictly medical framework, and highly constrained by social acceptability. So, for example, a woman experiencing infertility because of blocked tubes will be told that medicine can help by either unblocking the tubes or bypassing them (through IVF): other, social, options are not part of this framework. Adoption, for example, offers a solution to some of the problems of infertility. Yet infertility (and fertility) are becoming increasingly medicalised, and the choice of non-medical solutions is becoming a less obvious option for women.

Doctors are, inevitably, less concerned with the social domain in which women experience fertility/infertility. They may have some influence over it – in encouraging a woman to seek genetic counselling, for example – but on the whole, doctors see it as outside of their sphere. They do, however, see biological processes as 'their' sphere, although the women whose bodies undergo those processes may see things differently. And it is these processes that doctors will seek to influence if a woman seeks their help to overcome infertility. But what we should bear in mind – however awful or awe-inspiring a development seems (depending on your view of reproductive technologies) – is that science is really not very good at altering the biological processes fundamentally.

The underlying biological processes of ovulation, fertilisation, implantation and pregnancy are, quite simply, too poorly understood for scientists to be able to exert much control over them. What doctors seek to do is either to prevent a process or to 'help' the body to carry out the process. So, if fertilisation is prevented by mechanical blockage, it can take place in the laboratory, outside the woman's body. But the fertilisation itself is not under direct medical control: the *process* by which it occurs is up to nature.

It is the processes, however, that can fail, and lead to infertility. There are, roughly, four steps in the biological events that can lead to problems with fertility:

1. *Insufficient eggs or sperm*. The first step towards normal fertility is the production of eggs and sperm. On average, a woman produces one mature egg per month, on a cyclical basis (see boxes 4.1 and 4.2); men produce sperm continuously. So, the first cause of infertility is a dearth of eggs or sperm. For example a woman may not regularly release mature eggs (ovulate), although she has ovaries that appear to contain eggs; or, she may fail to ovulate because she lacks ovaries altogether for some reason. Men may produce no sperm, or so few that the chance of any reaching an egg is small.
2. *Failure of conception*. The second process of reproduction is fertilisation itself, in which a sperm makes

contact with an egg and fuses with it. But to do so, they have to be able to meet; if they cannot, no fertilisation can take place. The commonest cause of this in women is that the Fallopian tubes are blocked for some reason: the egg cannot then get from the ovary to the womb, nor can sperm ascend the tube to reach the egg. Conception may fail, too, when a man produces sperm that are not very active: if most sperm cannot swim actively, then the chances of conception are slim.

3. *Failure to implant*. The third stage of reproduction is implantation. Once the egg has been fertilised, it continues down the woman's Fallopian tube and enters her uterus. At this stage it has progressed from a fertilised egg into being an embryo; by this time, it is a ball of cells, some of which will form the fetus and some the membranes that will surround the fetus. Once inside the uterus, it should begin to burrow into the uterine lining, a process known as implantation. A woman may be infertile because embryos fail to implant into her uterus; as a result, they cease to develop. This would happen if, for instance, the embryo moves through the reproductive tract too quickly for some reason, or arrives at the uterus before the uterine lining is quite ready.

4. *Failure of early pregnancy*. Once the embryo has implanted itself, it begins its development. It has now to produce its membranes, and begin to develop its internal organs (its heart, brain and so on). Once these have begun to develop, the embryo becomes a fetus. But at this stage early miscarriage may occur, which can be just as stressful and disheartening an experience as a failure to conceive. That is, an embryo may implant itself in the wall of the uterus and begin to develop, but subsequently die, perhaps because of some genetic defect. This often happens so early that

the woman may not even know she had been pregnant. Or, the embryo may be genetically normal, but miscarry slightly later in pregnancy for unknown reasons. One such cause is a condition that doctors call 'incompetent cervix', when, for some reason, the woman's cervix opens slightly and provokes miscarriage. Most fertilised eggs probably fail to become viable pregnancies, so spontaneous abortion can be classed as a form of infertility only when a woman miscarries frequently. (Stillbirths – that is, death of the fetus after twenty-eight weeks of pregnancy – are, fortunately, rare now. If a baby is stillborn because of some genetic defect, there is a chance that a subsequent pregnancy will be affected. Women to whom this happens would not normally be classed as subfertile, but may turn to some forms of reproductive technology, such as embryo transfer, in order to have a baby while avoiding the risk of the genetic defect.)

In this, and the subsequent two chapters, we will deal with these 'failures' in the biological processes, and discuss what can be done in each case. For each, we will outline what is happening to the biological processes, and how they may fail; we will also outline how the medical profession sees the problems and what it seeks to do to solve them. Much of the biological detail is in boxes, ancillary to the main text, and provides background information. But our main discussion centres on the problems – ethical and social – raised by the interventions that women may have to face. In particular, many of these raise questions for feminists, about how we should respond to particular details of reproductive technologies and the medical context in which women usually have to confront them.

In some ways what the causes of infertility are may not matter much to a woman who wants a baby; her experience is a failure to conceive. Sometimes the reason may be obvious and sometimes less so. Nearly all women facing infertility will turn to doctors (there are few other choices; adoption, for instance, is increasingly difficult now). Once women have done so, their experience becomes increasingly shaped by medical decisions and diagnoses. Dealing with the experience of a failure to conceive because of blocked tubes, is different from the experience of finding out that your male partner does not produce enough sperm.

The four categories we have outlined are approximate, and infertility may in practice arise from several causes simultaneously. Clinicians attempting to 'cure' infertility attempt to establish where the problem lies biologically and then to treat it accordingly. The first step in medical diagnosis of infertility problems is to locate the cause. But focusing on the biological processes means that medics seek the *immediate* cause – failure to produce enough eggs or sperm, for example.

Yet by doing so other, less immediate causes are overlooked. What was it that caused someone to produce too few eggs/sperm? Or to suffer from blocked tubes? Sometimes these questions cannot be answered: if a man is infertile because he consistently produces sperm that are misshapen, that may be a quirk of his individual physiology. But it may also be because his work exposes him to dangerous chemicals or radiation, say, that damage the developing sperm. Similarly, a woman may have blocked tubes because of a previous infection, or because of prior surgery. Or, she may fail to ovulate because she is under stress or is underweight.

Doctors do sometimes take these less immediate causes into account; they may, for example, prefer that a woman gains weight before referring her to infertility treatment. And men with a low sperm count may be encouraged to wear less tight clothing to reduce the temperature of their testes. But, on the whole, a woman seeking medical help is more likely to find that doctors aim to treat the immediate problem.

The first, immediate cause of infertility, may be that there are simply not enough eggs or sperm produced. Why should this happen? The final stage of production of mature eggs and sperm depends upon certain hormones. It might fail if, for instance, the cocktail of hormones is not well co-ordinated, or if the levels of a particular hormone are low. So, one common form of treatment for infertility in a woman involves trying to correct any hormone problems so that she can produce mature eggs for fertilisation. Men, too, may fail to produce effective sperm for hormonal reasons, or because their testes fail to produce live sperm.

There are few choices for women who fail to ovulate because of low hormone levels. If they have cause to believe that stress is a reason for the low hormone levels, they may prefer to wait until a less stressful period of their lives. They may prefer to see if alternative treatments, such as homeopathy or acupuncture, can do anything for them. But the only reliable way of changing hormone levels is through hormonal drugs: it is also the quickest. As a treatment for infertility, hormonal drugs work only for some women who have particular kinds of hormone deficiency. From the medical point of view, the difficulty lies in deciding whether the problem *will* be solved by a hormonal drug. From a woman's point of view problems arise when women are sometimes given hormones when they don't need them, either because diagnosis was incorrect or as a last-ditch attempt by a doctor to do something.

But suppose that a woman has had the infertility diagnosed as resulting from a hormone deficiency; she has a reproductive system that appears structurally normal, but she simply produces too little of a particular hormone. What happens then? The obvious answer would seem to be to give her more of the hormone. That is one method, but it is not the only one. There are two other ways of boosting a woman's hormones medically. One is to make the woman's own body secrete more hormones (e.g. by stimulating the systems that control the production of her hormones); another is to 'trick' the body into acting as though there are more hormones present than there actually are (e.g. by altering the body's sensitivity to hormones).

Perhaps the commonest type of infertility treatment aims to alter levels of the hormones, the gonadotrophins, that control what the ovaries do, and thus stimulate ovulation. Roughly one-fifth of all women experiencing infertility are not ovulating for some hormonal reason, and are likely to be offered hormone treatment. A direct way of doing this is for the doctor to give the woman injections of gonadotrophins, which in turn stimulate her ovaries to produce eggs. One of these, for instance, is the drug Pergonal, which has also been used in conjunction with IVF.

Until recently, one of the commonest drugs used to boost gonadotrophins indirectly – and hence induce ovulation – was a drug called clomiphene (Clomid). Clomiphene works by sticking to the cells of the body that would normally become attached to oestrogen making oestrogen less able to affect those cells even though there is plenty of it around. The cells in the brain respond to this apparent lack of oestrogen by producing *more* of their hormones, the gonadotrophins. In turn, these stimulate the ovaries to produce more eggs (see boxes 4.1 and 4.2 for explanation of the biology involved).

Although making less oestrogen available to the brain is just what clomiphene has been asked to do, it sometimes does it too well. Other parts of the body actually need oestrogens for them to work properly and make pregnancy happen. So, although clomiphene makes about 70 to 80 per cent of women who take it ovulate, only about a third of these women actually go on to establish a pregnancy. The rest ovulate – but, because of the lack of oestrogen, the cells of their cervix (the neck of the womb) fail to produce enough mucus to allow the sperm to swim through into the womb. Newer drugs, such as Rehibin (cyclofenil) are less potent – and so may avoid the undesirable side effects.

What can be done when infertility is due to the man not producing enough sperm, and the problem facing the woman is still how to achieve a pregnancy? In principle, she could get round the problem and achieve fertilisation by using

Box 4.1 *Producing Eggs 1*

The first requirement for conception is that a woman produces healthy eggs. Even before she is born, a female's ovaries contain many cells that are destined to become eggs. But, in order for an adult woman to conceive, these potential eggs have to be made mature, a process which our bodies achieve using hormones. So producing eggs requires two things, either of which could be impaired in women who are infertile: first, a woman needs to have potential egg cells, and second, she needs to have an adequate supply of hormones.

What happens if a woman lacks potential eggs? This happens very rarely, when a female is born without ovaries. If, as an adult, she wants to have a child, then she will have to 'borrow' either an egg or possibly a live baby. This used to mean either adoption of a baby or surrogacy of some kind (for example, by means of her partner inseminating another woman who carried the baby to term). This is particularly controversial, and so she may prefer to 'borrow' an egg directly. This is possible only if she has a uterus: doctors could then take an egg from another woman and inseminate it with sperm from the partner of the woman lacking ovaries. Provided she then has hormone treatments to maintain the pregnancy, doctors could then implant the embryo into her uterus.

Hormone treatments are more commonly used to bring eggs to maturity. Newspaper reports used to refer to these as 'fertility drugs', though this is a bit of a misnomer. There are many different kinds of hormone treatment, each of which aims to correct a particular malfunction in the complex hormonal controls by which reproduction operates. Most women who are infertile and receive hormone treatments will receive them for this purpose. So, the purpose of the treatment is to ensure that a woman's body actually brings some eggs to maturity, so that they could be fertilised. But hormone treatments are also used in conjunction with IVF, to ensure an *excess* of mature eggs. Most women who undergo IVF can

(*Continued overleaf*)

produce mature eggs normally, but are infertile because their Fallopian tubes are blocked. IVF aims to bypass the blockage by removing eggs and fertilising them outside the body.

So, there are, roughly, three ways in which doctors and scientists can, at present, intervene to change the rate at which mature eggs are available so that a woman can bear a child. These are: 1. They can take mature eggs from *another* woman, and use them to enable women to become pregnant who produce no eggs at all. 2. They can increase the chances of a woman producing eggs that are properly mature, by hormones. 3. They can similarly use hormones to produce *extra* eggs, so that enough are fertilised to put into a woman's body for IVF.

Box 4.2 *Producing Eggs 2: Manipulating Numbers*

The key to altering a woman's egg production is hormones. The potential egg cells in her ovaries have, if they are to become eggs, to undergo two processes. First, they have to be 'matured': that is, they have to grow and to surround themselves with a protective envelope. Second, being mature is not enough: they have also to be pushed out of the ovary, so that they can travel along the Fallopian tube. The egg's protective envelope is important at this stage because it seems to help sperm to fuse with the egg, and also to help the Fallopian tube to move it along.

Both of these stages are achieved by hormones. Hormone controls in reproduction are very complex, and scientists do not understand them fully. There are broadly three components to it, all of which could 'malfunction' in a woman who cannot conceive. Ovaries are stimulated by hormones (called gonadotrophins) produced by the pituitary gland at the base of your brain. But ovaries do not just produce eggs: they also produce their own hormones (such as oestrogens). So, as pituitary hormones stimulate ovaries, the ovaries respond by producing mature eggs *and* more hormones.

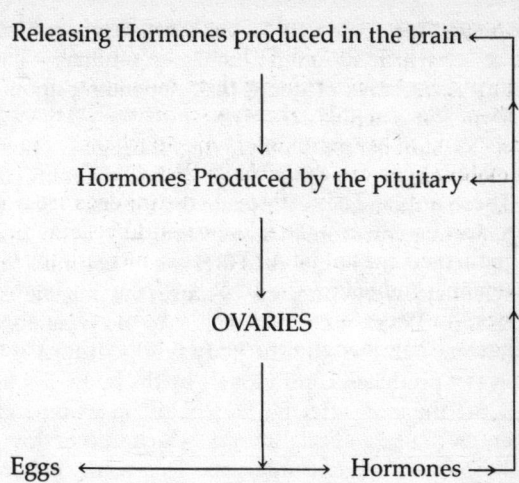

The arrows on the right of the diagram indicate controls. That is, the amount of hormones secreted by the ovaries helps to control the amount of hormones produced by the brain, which in turn controls those produced by the pituitary . . . and so on.

So what can doctors do if a woman is infertile because of something not working properly in these hormone controls? Hormones from the ovaries themselves are not particularly important for fertilisation itself; after all, if a woman's ovaries are working well enough to produce eggs at all, then they are likely to produce hormones too – although of course if any one stage of this control is not working properly, then it will probably have effects on the other stages. The first job a doctor has to do is to distinguish whether a component is not working properly because of something wrong within itself (something wrong with the pituitary, say) or it is not working because whatever controls it is not working.

The most critical stages for *producing* eggs are the first two, since it is pituitary hormones that make eggs mature and make the ovaries release them. Most women who are treated

(*Continued overleaf*)

> by hormones (approximately 80 per cent) are given hormones similar to, or which stimulate, their own pituitary. There are several different ways of doing this, depending upon where the malfunction is actually occurring.
>
> A smaller number of women might be given hormones similar to those in the first stage of the diagram; that is, hormones that themselves stimulate the pituitary. But it is not enough just to give a woman an injection, say, of the hormone (the most important is called LHRH – e.g. Fertiral): to begin with, scientists were puzzled because the injections were unsuccessful. What they had failed to do was to mimic accurately enough the way the body works. It turns out that LHRH is not produced continuously by the body, but in short 'pulses'. So, the most effective way of giving a woman LHRH treatment is to use a special pump, which injects tiny pulses of the hormone at regular intervals. This works better – and at a much tinier dose of the hormone.
>
> Some of these hormone treatments provoke the ovary to produce *more* than one mature egg, so twins and multiple pregnancies are relatively common. Doctors have decreased the risk of this, by giving women lower doses of the hormones – though the risk remains. Still, producing 'extra' eggs at any ovulation, with exact timing, is precisely what doctors aim to do with hormone treatments used in IVF and GIFT (Gamete Intra Fallopian Transfer). The aim is to produce several mature eggs so that at least two or three fertilised embryos can be reimplanted into the woman, so giving her a greater chance of pregnancy. So, the hormone treatments preceding egg removal are designed to make a woman 'superovulate' – that is, produce more than one egg – ideally, without stimulating the ovaries too much (which can make a woman ill).

sperm from someone else. Many women faced with this, however, would prefer to find ways of conceiving using their partner's sperm: again, that usually means seeking medical advice.

Men may be infertile for various reasons: because they

produce too few, or no sperm, or if the sperm fail to get to the egg (e.g. sperm that are badly shaped are less able to swim through the woman's reproductive tract). More rarely, they may be infertile because of something going wrong with ejaculation (ejaculation may not occur, or the sperm may be ejected backwards into the man's reproductive tract).

One of the more common causes of impaired fertility in men is temperature: if, for any reason, a man's testes are subjected to too high a temperature, the production of sperm slows down. Some men can deal with this problem by simply wearing looser clothing. Another cause is a kind of varicose vein in the testis, called a varicocele: as this vein becomes blocked up with blood, it gets hotter, thus impairing sperm production. Like varicose veins, it can be removed surgically.

Other treatments designed to increase numbers of sperm usually involve hormones. For instance, a man may be producing too few sperm because he is producing too little gonadotrophin. Gonadotrophins are sometimes given to men in an attempt to increase sperm count. The side effects are perhaps less severe than they are in women, or at least less life-threatening than, say, ectopic pregnancy (i.e. pregnancy occurring in sites other than the uterus – the Fallopian tubes, for example), though they do include bloating and slight breast growth, which many men may be unwilling to tolerate. On the other hand, hormone treatments for male infertility have tended to be a rather hit-or-miss affair, since there is, as yet, little good evidence that any of them actually do increase the supply of sperm.

Doctors have tried, for instance, giving infertile men injections of gonadotrophins, or of clomiphene, in efforts to increase the sperm yield. These may work in a few cases, although the treatment often has to be continued over several months if sperm yield is to increase significantly: this is for the simple reason that, unlike eggs, sperm are produced continuously and it takes at least seventy days for mature sperm to develop.

One reason why hormone treatments for men are so hit-or-miss is simply that there has been less research into the ways that hormones control male reproductive processes – partly due, no doubt, to the widespread belief that it is women rather than men that suffer from 'barrenness'. Another reason may be that the treatments used have not been appropriate. Until recently, doctors usually treated men who were subfertile for some hormonal reason with either gonadotrophins or with the hormones that themselves stimulate gonadotrophins, the releasing hormones (e.g., GnRH – Gonadotrophin Releasing Hormone: this stimulates gonadotrophin, which in turn stimulates the testes). Because these control gonadotrophins, doctors reasoned, injecting them ought to make the body increase its output of gonadotrophins and in turn provoke the testes into producing more sperm. Unfortunately, the patients' gonadotrophins did not respond as planned: if anything, they declined after a time.

What the doctors had not realised was that hormones like GnRH are not released continuously, but in pulses every ninety minutes or so (in both women and men). For these treatments to work, they have to simulate exactly the way that the body works: doctors can now do this through tiny pumps attached to the person's body. This pulsatile treatment has worked in a small proportion of men and women who are infertile because of problems with the hormones produced by the brain (see box 4.2) and a few have achieved pregnancy. One other important advantage of treatments like this is that the doses of GnRH are very small. So, unpleasant side effects are less likely.

Understanding how GnRH controls gonadotrophins has led to a new form of treatment for women's infertility that, paradoxically, involves *reducing* gonadotrophin levels. Doctors have recently begun to use a drug that mimics GnRH, called buserelin. At first, as expected, buserelin stimulates the body to produce more gonadotrophin – but the levels then decline. GnRH in our bodies is normally produced in pulses, allowing enough time in between pulses for the cells secreting gonadotrophin to recover. Continuous buserelin treatment 'wears out' these cells temporarily; so, gonadotrophin levels eventually decline.

Buserelin is also useful for treating women whose infertility is the result of polycystic ovary disease. Women with cystic ovaries have a high level of one of the gonadotrophins which probably interferes with ovulation. So, giving these women a drug that reduces their levels of gonadotrophin can help them to become pregnant. Another medical use of buserelin is in conjunction with IVF. In this case, what doctors are aiming to do is to 'switch off' the woman's own gonadotrophins. They do this partly because they believe that, in some cases of infertility, the woman's production of hormones is faulty; and partly because giving the woman an injection of gonadotrophins gives them greater control over the process of egg production. This, the doctors believe, allows them to time the injections more precisely. At any rate, some studies suggest that using buserelin leads to a greater success rate in pregnancies achieved on IVF programmes than if gonadotrophins were used alone.[1]

Though the mechanisms are complicated, the aim of all such treatments is to achieve ovulation – the production of a fertile egg. If this happens, and a pregnancy results, then most women would feel it was worth it. But, like many forms of medical treatment, many of these hormonal treatments do not come without a price: apart from all the practical problems of attending clinics and monitoring a woman's hormones, most of the drugs have some side effects. Pamphlets produced by the manufacturers of some of these treatments warn, for instance, of the risks of 'ovarian hyperstimulation', ectopic pregnancies and multiple pregnancies resulting from stimulation of gonadotrophins. That these 'fertility drugs' can provoke multiple pregnancies has been known for some time, and medical reports have recently begun to emphasise the need to monitor the dose carefully to minimise such risks. Even so, monitoring may not always work: the tragedy of the Halton septuplets, conceived as a result of hormone treatments, who were born three months prematurely, but who subsequently died, is one example.

Another problem for women taking 'fertility drugs' such as clomiphene is that they can feel ill: the side effects are similar to those experienced by some women at the menopause, such as nausea, flushing and abdominal bloating. Severe headaches and hair loss are also possible. One woman noted that she 'felt very ill' after taking clomiphene to promote ovulation and subsequently decided not to go on with infertility investigations.[2] Another had been taking clomiphene for months before she discovered that the trouble she had been having with her eyes probably resulted from the clomiphene.[3]

The newer treatments, like buserelin, probably pose less risk of multiple pregnancies, because, in principle, the timing and doses can be calculated with more precision. This is possible because drugs like buserelin alter gonadotrophin levels directly; earlier drugs did so indirectly, and it was not possible to predict with accuracy what quantities of gonadotrophin the body would produce in response to the drug. But buserelin is not without side effects either; reducing gonadotrophins leads to lower oestrogen levels, so women on buserelin sometimes experience symptoms similar to the menopause. Using buserelin, on the other hand, produces more pregnancies in IVF; for some women, the side effects may seem a small price to pay for pregnancy.

However, it has not, on the whole, been these kinds of hormonal treatments that have aroused controversy. If anything, hormone treatments for infertility have become quite unglamorous. There are two particular areas of controversy surrounding solutions to problems of too few eggs/sperm. First, women may seek a solution to male infertility through artificial insemination, or to their own lack of eggs by egg donation from another woman; both of these are suspect for many religious traditionalists because they take reproduction outside the nuclear family.

Second, what has aroused criticism from feminists and others are the more 'high-tech', high-profile procedures like IVF (discussed in more detail in the next chapter), with their implications of increased medical management of women's bodies (suppressing women's gonadotrophins only in order to give them by injection might be one example of such management, even if it does yield greater 'success' in terms of pregnancy). Yet we should remember that IVF, too, is based fundamentally on the *same* hormone treatments that have been around for some time. The principal difference is that IVF entails giving hormones in larger doses to women whose own hormones probably work perfectly well. The issue then is not one of getting a woman's body to produce any eggs at all, but of getting her to produce an excess of them.

Hormone treatments are given as part of infertility treatments for basically two reasons: to women who fail to ovulate and women undergoing IVF. The difference is that, in the first case, the role of the hormones is to induce relatively *normal* responses (a normal ovulation of one egg, for instance), while in the case of IVF, doctors hope to induce *higher than normal* responses. That is, to ensure that they will obtain enough eggs to fertilise in vitro, doctors want the woman's ovary to respond by producing *several* mature eggs at a time (see box 4.3).

Pushing the body's responses too far has its dangers, however, and women often find regimens of daily hormone injections stressful and difficult to fit into busy lives. Advertising pamphlets refer to the side effect of ovarian hyperstimulation – stimulating the ovaries rather more than is usual during a menstrual cycle. But what does hyperstimulation involve? Apart from what it does to the ovary's production of eggs, hyperstimulation does result, for some women, in nausea and abdominal discomfort. Yet again this, and the stresses of injections, may seem to many women to be worth putting up with because it offers the possibility of a much-wanted pregnancy.

Box 4.3 *How are Eggs Retrieved?*

Unlike sperm, eggs are produced inside a human body and so are difficult to get at. Normally fertile women who want to conceive have to try and predict the moment when their ovaries are releasing eggs (by, say, temperature change) and time insemination (natural or artificial) accordingly. Prediction is rather easier for women who are infertile but are being treated with hormones, since the timing of the hormones themselves give some clue about ovulation.

But for women whose infertility has some physical cause, such as blocked Fallopian tubes, the block has to be bypassed – which means removing eggs from the body. In IVF, they are then fertilised outside, in the laboratory, before being replaced. In GIFT, the eggs are mixed with the partner's sperm in the laboratory, and immediately replaced into the woman's tubes so that fertilisation occurs inside her body.

Actually retrieving eggs is not easy. There are enough technical difficulties in getting to a woman's ovaries to remove eggs – without subjecting her to large-scale surgery and stays in hospital. But, first, the eggs have to mature just at the right stage; so, the woman has initially to be given hormones to ripen her eggs. Using ultrasound scans, doctors can determine how big the ripening eggs are. Once they are big enough, she will be given another hormone to make the ovaries release the eggs. It is at precisely this moment that they have to be retrieved. There are, currently, two methods of doing this: the first, and commonest, method is laparoscopy. The disadvantage of this method is that the woman has to be anaesthetised, since it requires inserting a fine, hollow needle through her abdomen; this can be guided using ultrasound scanners, to the surface of the ovary, from which the eggs are sucked out gently one by one.

Newer methods do not need full anaesthesia, and so are more likely to become available in out-patient departments. One of these is called TUDOR (trans-vesicle, ultrasound-directed oocyte recovery). This requires only local anaesthesia, with a suction needle inserted through the bladder, from the woman's vagina.

How Many Eggs Are Enough? The Risks to Women

Feminist criticism has, on the whole, centred either on the general effects of all interventions in reproduction, or has dealt specifically with the use of hormones to produce an excess of eggs. One controversy has centred on the possibility that the practice of deliberately increasing the supply of eggs might lead to women's bodies being used specifically for that purpose.

Most feminists would agree that the context in which women reproduce and in which new technologies are generated is patriarchal. Most doctors are men – and they are likely to be white and middle-class – so that the doctor–woman patient relationship is intrinsically one of power imbalance in this society. Women, moreover, are the reproducers of life – one important reason why they come into greater contact with medical professionals than do men. But this greater contact has also come to involve increasingly extensive management of women's role in reproduction. Ann Oakley has noted that, in earlier decades of this century, the major objective of obstetric intervention was to preserve the life of the mother: bearing children was still a fairly risky business, and the mother's life may be at stake. But things have changed: she comments that '. . . as the risks encountered by women in childbearing became less in the 1950s, mothers gradually began to acquire within the medical perspective a new guise as containers of fetuses'.[4] It is in this context that medical interventions which aim to make women ovulate must be assessed.

As we have seen, part of the power of doctors lies in deciding what information will be given out, and to whom. The woman who suffered severe eye problems while taking clomiphene was, evidently, not told that there might be side effects.[5] Feminists have often noted that women are sometimes not told of the risks attached to taking hormonal drugs – the injectable contraceptive, Depo-Provera,[6] for example, or of possible risks of taking hormones for years after the menopause.

The tendency to withhold information from at least some women stems partly from the kind of misogyny that Hilary Graham and Ann Oakley found in the research they did on the behaviour of doctors towards women in antenatal clinics. Apart from trivialising women's anxieties, doctors also tend to disbelieve women, to assume ignorance – even to the extent of checking a woman's medical notes in one case because the doctor did not believe the mother's own assertion that her previous children had both been girls.[7] Graham and Oakley cite one doctor, irritated by a woman asking further questions about induction, who said: 'If we explained to everyone, and everyone's husband, we'd spend all our time explaining. *I think you've got to assume if you come here for medical attention that we make all the decisions*. In fact, I think you should come in today, but I've already been browbeaten into saying Sunday, which is another forty-eight hours.'[8]

Given such attitudes, women are often not going to be given full information about the risks to health – theirs or that of the fetus. For instance, when a woman who has no ovaries conceives (as a result of IVF), she has to be given hormonal drugs for some weeks afterwards in order to maintain the pregnancy. Thus, the fetus is also being continuously exposed to these hormones.

Critics of IVF, including some feminists, have drawn a historical parallel with a drug called diethylstilboestrol (DES). It was used in the 1940s to prevent miscarriages, particularly in the US with terrible long-term consequences for the fetus exposed to it while in the uterus. What emerged much later was that the daughters and sons of mothers who received DES suffered from rare forms of cancer after puberty (vaginal adenocarcinoma in women, and scrotal carcinoma in men). DES is a good example of how powerful some drugs can be in causing damage before birth, just as thalidomide was. But it is a bad example for feminists to use when arguing against doctors' use of hormones because the doctors do not consider it to be a 'natural' hormone. That is, it is synthetic (i.e. manufactured in the laboratory) and a molecule of DES is not quite the same as the hormones it mimics, in other words, it is not actually an oestrogen, although it has many properties that are *like* that of oestrogen.

Doctors who defend the use of hormones emphasise that 'natural' hormones – hormones that are chemically identical to those produced by our bodies – can be used more safely for anything from menopausal problems to the maintenance of pregnancy. But safety is difficult to evaluate and there may well be more subtle, long-term effects of taking hormones that are not produced by one's own body. The fetus, especially during the first weeks, is particularly vulnerable; there are certainly data from research using animals that show all kinds of effects of early exposure to hormones, including apparent masculinisation of female fetuses, and in mother's milk on the reproductive hormones of the offspring. The babies born to those women given hormones during IVF appear to be healthy, but they are only infants, and the numbers are small.

We may not know in detail what long-term consequences there are if fetuses are exposed to hormones: but we do know that one consequence of hormone treatments for infertility is sometimes multiple pregnancies. The risk of this can be greater when IVF is used, just because doctors often return several embryos to a woman's womb to increase the chances of pregnancy. Multiple pregnancies may be desirable for some women seeking infertility treatment; as one woman put it, 'I'd got so excited about the [hormone treatment] because one of the side effects is to have multiple births. I thought that was fantastic, a whole family at once. It was the first real hope we'd had.'[9]

At present, the chances of becoming pregnant if only one egg is fertilised in vitro and returned to the woman are small – ten per cent at most[10]. Doctors working on IVF programmes generally agree that two or more fertilised eggs should be put back into the woman's body in order to increase the chances: but there has been vehement disagreement over just how many. The Voluntary Licensing Authority, which issues guidelines in Britain for IVF work, insists that usually no more than three eggs should be replaced, although a few doctors continued for a while to replace more just to increase the chances of pregnancy.

Yet multiple pregnancies do carry greater risk to the woman's health, and also a greater chance of miscarrying. If carried to term, they can also impose enormous financial and social burdens. Realising that she has a multiple pregnancy may well evoke very mixed feelings towards the pregnancy: however much she wanted the pregnancy, it may be hard to face having three or more babies at once.

One medical response to the problem of multiple pregnancy is to reduce the number of fetuses that the woman is carrying. Doctors can do this by cardiac puncture – by a needle to pierce the fetal heart. The rest of the fetuses may go through an uneventful pregnancy – though the risks are high. Approximately fifty per cent of women undergoing the procedure miscarry altogether. Although not widely practised, that selective reduction is possible has provoked controversy about its ethics. Not surprisingly, anti-abortion agencies are horrified: Nuala Scarisbrook, administrator of Life argued that 'If a woman wants to have a baby she should do what women have always done and accept what comes. Having found she [a woman in Holland] was expecting quins, she should have carried on'.[11]

Multiple pregnancies are very risky to a woman's health; there is, for instance, a much greater risk of severe haemorrhage and high blood pressure. Indeed, doctors are developing one form of selective reduction specifically to safeguard the mother's life. Both ectopic and multiple pregnancies are more common after techniques like IVF; occasionally, both occur together. A woman might, for instance, have one embryo implanted normally in her uterus, and another ectopically in her Fallopian tube. Ectopic pregnancies threaten a woman's life, and so have to be ended: but, most surgical techniques for doing so will also threaten the survival of the embryo in the womb. So doctors are now trying to find a method of destroying the ectopic embryo by injecting it directly with a drug to poison it (ultrasound allows them to do this fairly precisely) with less risk to the embryo in the womb. We can only guess at how distressed a woman would feel after going through so much – infertility investigations, and procedures that result in the overproduction of eggs – only to be told on finding herself pregnant that she should have some of the fetuses punctured or poisoned to reduce the risks to the pregnancy.

Apart from risks to health, multiple pregnancies, if all the babies survive, also pose huge problems of care and money. After all the publicity has died down, mothers of five or more usually find that they no longer get the free 'hand outs' from commercial companies keen to sponsor their baby products. And they also find that welfare benefits are hopelessly inadequate. Moreover, most fetuses in multiple pregnancies are born prematurely, and have to have intensive care for many weeks, thus putting great strain on regional neonatal units, which in turn can prevent other premature babies from getting the attention they need.

Unless techniques are improved so that there is a better chance of pregnancy with only one egg replaced after IVF, the risk of multiple pregnancy will remain, along with the risk to health and the associated ethical questions. Still, it is not only questions of the risk to health posed by multiple pregnancies that concern feminists. Some feminist writers have also stressed that the increasing medical management of reproduction in general means greater control by men over women and their bodies. In this regard, one aspect that is causing concern is the removal and donation of eggs: that eggs can be removed from women's bodies may mean that it becomes possible to do so without a woman's consent or even knowledge. There is always the possibility that doctors might be involved in coercing women into 'donating' eggs, either for research or to donate to other women.

The Warnock Committee deliberated over the ethics of egg

donation, and concluded that it should be considered acceptable as a means of alleviating infertility (i.e. eggs being donated by a fertile woman to an infertile one), while recognising the risks to the donor from surgery and possible unwanted pregnancy. But these disadvantages should be weighed, the committee felt, against the benefits: 'For some couples egg donation provides the only chance of their having a child which the woman can carry to term, and which is the genetic child of her husband'.[12]

Women themselves are not necessarily antagonistic towards the idea of donating eggs, even for research. Elizabeth Alder and her colleagues reported on a study of the attitudes of women attending antenatal and family planning clinics in Edinburgh, towards IVF and embryo research.[13] One of the questions the women were asked was whether or not they thought that women should be allowed to donate eggs for research. The researchers found that more than 70 per cent of the women interviewed said they thought women should be allowed to do this, and more than 60 per cent said they might be willing to donate eggs themselves. So, although the question was not phrased in quite these terms, the women in the sample presumably did not feel that donating eggs was necessarily always 'bad for women': egg harvesting for research might, after all, help other women in the future.

Still, the procedures do involve risks to the health of the donor, and there is a danger that women who donate are not fully informed of available choices. Not all women, moreover, would be willing to donate eggs for research, although they might be happy to donate eggs to a specific recipient. These risks do raise questions for feminist analysis.

The most important issue that these procedures raise is the possibility of enhanced medical control over patients. One risk is that doctors will select which women are most 'suitable' to be donors. White, middle-class, married women are more likely to be selected, just as they are more likely to be treated for infertility. Another way in which control is enhanced is that the donor is brought into a *medical* framework. Although some women may donate eggs while they themselves are undergoing some form of treatment, others may not; a woman may decide, for example, to donate eggs to another woman after she has had her own, uneventful, pregnancy. Once she had made that decision, she enters the medical domain.

Clearly, some of the issues raised in feminist critiques – such as male control over women as patients – cut across many aspects of women's health. Some are more specific, either to reproductive technologies in general (the issues that infertility raises for our experience as women) or to forms of intervention (e.g. health risks due to hormones). The use of hormones alone to alleviate infertility is less often mentioned in critiques, even though it is the foundation for the 'superovulation' that is necessary to IVF. Somehow, because the *kind* of intervention (injection with hormones) is not new (though different forms of hormones are), this form of reproductive control seems sometimes to be overshadowed by the higher-technology versions like IVF. But the issues it raises remain.

The most salient questions for feminism, as far as techniques for producing eggs and sperm are concerned, seem to be these: first, how can we assess, and if necessary gain some control over, the use of hormones in promoting fertility? We need to make this assessment not only in relation to IVF, but also to the more widespread applications of hormone technology. Second, should we care about the number, or fate, of eggs (or sperm) that we produce? Some of the concern about the possibility of 'harvesting eggs' rests on the moral assumption that we have some rights over our gametes (eggs or sperm). It follows, then, that it is not morally acceptable for a society to use gametes in research or to remove them from people's bodies for any other purpose. One question that feminists need to address is whether we agree with this premise. Do we believe that our eggs are so much 'ours' that we have the right to donate them in a will as we might other life-giving organs? Eggs are, in some senses, part of the *next* generation – so what rights should we have, or not have, over them as individuals? These are questions we must deal with if we are to be able to resist challenges to our role in reproduction effectively.

5. Fertilisation and IVF

Life, it is said by some, begins at fertilisation. This belief is also at the centre of many ethical controversies currently raging over IVF. If life is said to begin at fertilisation, then a fertilised egg in the laboratory is equivalent to a human embryo growing in a woman's uterus: if one should be accorded special protection, say critics, so should the other.

The question of when life begins has troubled theologians for centuries. In the Middle Ages, human life was widely believed to begin at the moment of 'quickening', when the mother first feels movements and the soul was said to have entered the fetal body (after about 80 days of gestation). But today, the 'beginning of life' has shifted; as we have seen in Chapter Three, many theologians now believe that human life begins at the moment of fertilisation and from that moment deserves special consideration.

Fertilisation is, for many critics of reproductive technology, the key moment of reproduction: it is, after all, the process in which egg and sperm combine and patterns of inheritance are determined. It is this belief that underlies the fears expressed by organisations like the Society for the Protection of Unborn Children (SPUC), about the fate of eggs fertilised in vitro. Most doctors are more likely, however, to treat implantation as the point at which life begins. Implantation is the moment at which the pregnancy starts, when the woman's body begins to behave differently; it is also the moment when recognisable changes occur that doctors can detect. For this reason, losing one or two potential embryos in the course of IVF arouses little medical consternation. Indeed, most fertilised eggs and early embryos that begin to develop after fertilisation occurs normally in the body, will fail to implant or to develop further. The 'natural' process is only a little less wasteful of embryos than the 'artificial' process of IVF.

The First Step: What is Fertilisation?

Fertilisation is the process whereby the sperm fuses with the egg and passes through its surface membrane, a process bringing in its wake a chain of chemical changes which alter the egg permanently. The most important changes it must undergo are, first, to make its surface membrane impermeable to any other sperm that may approach, and secondly, to begin the process of combining genetic material from the sperm with that from the egg.

Scientists worked out the basic principles of fertilisation in the late nineteenth century. But, a century later, there is still much that is unknown: they still argue, for instance, over just how the sperm actually penetrates the egg's surface (for details, see box 5.1). Because egg and sperm are so small, it is virtually impossible to observe fertilisation occurring in a living body, and very difficult to try to control it. Doctors can, as we have seen, try to encourage a woman to ovulate, and she can ensure that sperm are available at the right time, whether by intercourse or by artificial insemination. But the rest, the fertilisation itself, is up to nature.

Sometimes, though, nature does not co-operate. Because it is so hard to study fertilisation in its natural setting, no one knows whether some instances of infertility may result from a failure of fertilisation itself (for instance, because healthy egg and sperm meet, but somehow fail to combine). What doctors have more idea about is infertility that results from egg and sperm failing to meet in the first place, even though enough are produced. Basically, the blockage could be of two

Box 5.1. *What is Fertilisation?*

School biology textbooks conjure up images of active little sperm, swimming vigorously and burrowing their way into a passive egg, and that it is the sperm that uniquely determines the sex of the offspring. These images are only partly true.

First, at the point at which sperm are ejaculated, they are not capable of fertilising an egg. To do that, they have to be specially prepared (a process called sperm capacitation) by the internal secretions of the female's reproductive system. No one quite knows why or how capacitation works, although scientists have learned how to mimic it in vitro, so that fertilisation can occur in the lab (for this, the sperm have to be washed free of semen and put into a salt and nutrient solution). The secretions of the female's reproductive system, too, probably affect the rate at which sperm move: since Y-bearing sperm (that would produce male offspring) are lighter than X-bearing sperm (for female offspring), the chemical state of the female system probably influences which sperm actually get as far as the egg.

Second, in order to be able to penetrate an egg, the outside membrane of the sperm has to fuse with that of the egg; once that has happened, it is *not* all down to the thrusting sperm. Rather, the egg has actively to engulf the sperm, and 'help' it to enter.

The first step in fusing is that capacitation causes the outer layer of the sperm head to break down, as soon as it contacts the egg. It has to do this, or it will not be able to penetrate the outer layer (the zona) of the egg. As it breaks down, it releases chemicals that cause changes to occur in the structure of the zona; this in turn allows the sperm to penetrate through to the egg below (assisted at this point by its moving tail). Then, when it makes contact with the egg surface, the two membranes combine, and the sperm head is drawn into the egg. Once inside, something inhibits the sperm from further movement. Meanwhile, the egg starts to push out tiny granules from its surface: these, in turn, prevent any more sperm from entering the egg.

(*Continued overleaf*)

> Once inside, the chromosomes (containing all the genetic information) of sperm and egg combine, and then divide. As they divide, so too does the egg. It divides into two cells, then four, eight, sixteen and so on, and then into a tiny ball of cells. It is at this stage that it would be transferred into a woman's body during in vitro fertilisation.

kinds: it could be a chemical block that inhibits the movement of either egg or sperm, or it could be a mechanical block to the path of the egg, say (see box 5.2).

So what can women do when fertilisation fails? There are, roughly, three ways of approaching the problem: first, fertilisation may fail because the quality of sperm the man produces is poor (there may be a high proportion of misshapen or chemically abnormal sperm, for instance), or because the sperm cannot get past the woman's cervix. If fertilisation fails to take place because of problems with the quality or quantity of the man's sperm, the woman (or the couple) may choose to opt for artificial insemination. Or, if medical help is sought, a doctor may try giving the man hormones. Second, if the fertilisation fails because there is a physical blockage in the woman's reproductive system, and if she wants to bear her own child rather than, say, adopt, doctors can try to remove the blockage itself by drug treatment or surgery (see box 5.3). Third, if the first two approaches do not work, doctors can get round the problem of the blockage by making fertilisation take place outside the body (as in IVF and embryo transfer).

Artificial Insemination

One reason why fertilisation may fail is because a woman's cervix is producing mucus that prevents sperm from entering her uterus, or is producing antibodies that kill the sperm. If she seeks medical help, doctors may try to alter her chemistry

Box 5.2. *The Path of the Egg: Transport*

Once it has left the ovary, the egg has to make its way towards the uterus (womb). The ovary is only partially attached to the Fallopian tube, and the egg might be released anywhere on the surface of the ovary. So, to get *into* the end of the tube, it has to be propelled towards it. At the end of the tube are tiny 'fingers', called fimbriae; these are covered with tiny moving hairs. As these move, they set up a current of fluid. Muscular movements of the tube and the adjacent ovary help maintain this flow, and the egg is wafted along towards the entrance to the tube.

Because of this fluid flow, eggs can be transported from an ovary on one side of the body, to the Fallopian tube on the other: women who have a blocked tube on one side, and no ovary on the other, have become pregnant, for instance, as a result of this. The egg, presumably, leaves the intact ovary, floats into the fluid-filled spaces in the woman's abdomen, and is picked up by the current created by the tube and its fimbriae on the opposite side. Knowing this has enabled doctors to develop a new technique called POST (Peritoneal Ovum–Sperm Transfer – the transfer of both egg and sperm directly into a woman's abdomen). This technique might be used, for instance, with women whose infertility is unexplained, or which is perhaps due to her cervix rejecting the sperm. It involves taking an unfertilised egg (obtained by laparoscopy) and some of her partner's sperm, mixing them in a suitable nutrient solution, and putting them into the woman's abdominal cavity (rather than in any specific part of her reproductive system, as in the GIFT technique (see box 4.2).

As the egg leaves the ovary, it is surrounded by a thin layer of cells called cumulus ('cloud-like') cells. These cells provide a kind of rough surface, against which the tiny hairs of the fimbriae, and inside the tube, can move. This, and muscular pushes from the tube, propel the egg along the first part of the tube; and, as it moves, its outer cumulus coat gets rubbed off. Twenty-four hours after it has left the ovary, the egg

(Continued overleaf)

usually arrives at the narrower part of the tube (the isthmus): here, there are fewer hairs, and the muscular movement tends to push it to and fro for a while (about another forty-eight hours). Eventually, however, it gets pushed rapidly towards the uterus.

Hormones can influence all these stages. Once the egg has left the ovary, it leaves a 'scar' behind that secretes the hormone progesterone. This has the effect of reducing the amount of movement that the uterus undergoes. So, if the egg is fertilised and begins to embed itself into the uterus, it is not pushed out immediately. Oestrogens, on the other hand, tend to make the reproductive tract *more* mobile. This is probably what happens with 'morning-after' pills, which contain high doses of oestrogens. If any eggs have been fertilised, the oestrogen makes the muscle of the tubes more active, so moving the fertilised egg along too fast for it to implant.

Box 5.3. *Fertilisation: What can go wrong?*

The three most likely kinds of chemical block are (i) the sperm cannot get through the cervix, perhaps because of the consistency of cervical mucus; (ii) the sperm get through but subsequently stick together; or (iii) the egg starts to break down before it can be fertilised. This can happen, for instance, because of a disease called endometriosis (see below).

The consistency of mucus is most likely to alter because of infection; if so, doctors will treat it with antibiotics. If sperm stick together after ejaculation, then it is probably because the man has produced antibodies to them; that is, his body's defences are behaving as though the sperm are invaders to be attacked. The woman's body, too, may produce antibodies to sperm, so that the sperm are killed after ejaculation. Sperm, of course, *are* invaders: they are not cells from the woman's body. (Curiously, though, most women's bodies do not normally attack sperm, for reasons that no one yet knows.) There isn't much that doctors can do about these responses: they might try giving that partner steroids, which suppress the body's defences (immune system). Occasionally, a pregnancy might result, but there is obviously a risk that the body can no longer effectively fight off disease.

Endometriosis is a painful condition, in which tiny pieces of the womb lining (endometrium) become attached to other parts of the abdomen – the intestines, for example. The endometrium normally secretes a hormone called prostaglandin, which makes the womb lining contract more forcefully. This is probably why endometriosis is painful. Prostaglandins may be the culprit in those women with this condition who are infertile; some doctors think that they interfere with the egg after it has left the ovary. Doctors usually prescribe hormone treatments for endometriosis: if that is the sole cause of a woman's infertility, then her chances of becoming pregnant after the treatment are about fifty per cent.

Mechanical blocks to fertilisation result most commonly from blocks in the Fallopian tubes, perhaps because of previous infection or because some other piece of tissue has stuck to the tube after surgery for some other condition (e.g. having an appendix out). Or, more rarely, doctors may find that a woman has a misshapen uterus. It is possible for doctors to correct some of these mechanical problems surgically, but not all: much depends upon the extent of the blockage. Surgery does improve the chances of pregnancy a little, although it also increases the chances of ectopic pregnancy (i.e. a pregnancy occurring outside of the uterus). But, if the tubes are very badly damaged, IVF may be the only option.

to make her cervix less hostile to sperm. For some women, hormone treatments may work, or antibiotics if the problem results from an infection. But another means of treating these problems is to bypass the cervix, using a form of artificial insemination. Artificial insemination, of course, is one answer to problems of infertility that need not involve medical intervention.

Still, doctors may recommend to a woman undergoing

infertility investigations that she try artificial insemination using her partner's sperm; this can sometimes help if the number of sperm is slightly low. The woman can do this herself, inserting the sperm high up in her vagina. If the doctor does it, he/she could either place the sperm into her cervix or inject it directly into her uterus by inserting a catheter through her cervix, thus bypassing any possible chemical blockage. Some doctors claim quite good success rates for this technique – 40 per cent in some cases[1] – others feel that there is little that can be done medically to overcome the problems posed, for example, by abnormal sperm.

Artificial insemination using a partner's sperm is not particularly controversial, and few doctors would hesitate to recommend it if they felt that it would solve the patient's problems. What is more controversial, however, is artificial insemination using donated sperm (artificial insemination by donor, or AID). Donating sperm is neither a particularly new technique, nor a 'high-tech' one, and AID may be the only solution for a woman who wants to bear her own child but whose partner cannot produce viable sperm.

So what are the problems? AID raises very different questions for feminists and those who would defend the status quo. AID is opposed by the Catholic Church partly because it separates procreation and sex. And many traditionalists oppose it because of their belief that a child has to be brought into a 'proper' family. One aspect of AID – especially if it is not subject to some form of regulation – that gives them cause for concern is the possibility that women living outside of conventional families could use it to have children. This, in turn, threatens to disrupt traditional ideas of patriarchal control and inheritance.

A related fear is that the widespread use of donated sperm might carry a risk of inbreeding. For example, it has been claimed that a woman seeking use of a frozen sperm sample from, say, a sperm bank might unwittingly use sperm from a man related to her, or that her children might end up producing children with their unknown half-siblings. But the probability of these mishaps is vanishingly small (except perhaps under odd special circumstances such as a sperm bank held by a small and already highly inbred group, such as some religious sects); clinics offering AID services tend to reduce these risks by restricting the number of times that a donor can be used.

Perhaps a more serious risk for those wishing to defend present social values is that a woman could choose to use sperm from someone who has died, an understandable response, perhaps, for someone recently bereaved, but still a response which challenges traditional patterns of inheritance. For that reason, the Warnock Report devoted a great deal of attention to it. A woman in France provoked controversy because she wanted to use sperm deposited in a sperm bank by her husband when he had had cancer diagnosed. When he eventually died, the woman requested his sperm to enable her to have his child. To some, the request was ghoulish; others emphasised the problems that could ensue with relatives over any estate. Does any resulting child automatically inherit from its father, however long ago that man died?

Another, more controversial, context in which AID is sometimes used is in relation to surrogacy; situations in which a woman is paid to carry a pregnancy to term for another couple, after being inseminated with the male partner's sperm. In the US, several lawsuits have followed claims that the paying couple have reneged on payments, or that the woman bearing the child has failed to hand it over. But contractual failures are not the only reason for controversy: much anger and fear is evoked by the woman who willingly carries a child in order to give it up, thus undermining, according to some, the stability of the family.

Yet what underlies all this concern with AID and 'proper' families is a more fundamental cause for alarm. AID – partly because it often involves sperm donated by a stranger – separates biological from social fatherhood. Because of that, it calls into question the inevitability and supposed 'naturalness' of current social arrangements, of patterns of inheritance in particular. For example, when it was revealed that lesbians had been using AID to have children the media howled with horror (lesbians with children have never had social support, often losing custody to fathers who had previously had little to do with the children). Any woman who attempts to raise children alone threatens the family and brings into question the status of fatherhood. But for women to make the separation of biological from social quite transparent by using AID was too much for conventional morality.

Inevitably, one result was a backlash, characterised by various attempts to restrict AID only to married, heterosexual couples. Several Christian organisations put forward cases to the Warnock Committee in relation to AID: the Christian Action Research and Education Trust, for instance, opposed AID (and many other interventions) on the grounds that 'every child has a right to be born the true child of a married couple'[2].

Feminists are, not surprisingly, less concerned with the stability of the nuclear family, or heterosexual marriage as an institution, and more with what happens to women. What has concerned feminists about the way that AID is practised in a medical context is the broader issue of power – doctors' power over women as 'patients' – and the issue of what might be termed 'quality control'. Maintaining sperm banks might, for instance, encourage the selection of specific donors on eugenic grounds, perhaps because of their ethnic background, or because of their specific qualities, or might lead to the selection of women recipients for their 'suitability'.

If sperm are used for AID, when it is practised in a medical context, then it is likely to be used only from 'approved' donors. Within the health services, the donors are often medics themselves. Ann Oakley describes increasing medical intervention in reproduction as a form of obstetric fatherhood, and comments:

> The patriarchal note in medical ideology has finally burst into the canon of obstetrical fatherhood – obstetricians are to

determine in this, as well as other ways, which women are to become mothers. As a matter of fact, there has been a surreptitious spreading of obstetrical fatherhood for some time in the vogue for using medical sperm in AID. Preferred donors for artificial insemination are English, middle-class, medical students . . . ; it is said (without evidence) that an acceptable level of intelligence, a stable personality, and character as a good 'all-rounder' is thereby assured.[3]

Not everyone would agree that stability and quality was thus assured, but this use of 'medical' sperm is an obvious attempt to select donors for their 'acceptable' characteristics.

Such selection attaches great importance to the role of genetics in determining the 'quality' of offspring, and has, at its most extreme, eugenic implications. If we select sperm donors on the basis of their qualities such as intelligence, it has been argued, those qualities will be passed on to the offspring and we can breed better quality people. William Shockley, who won a Nobel Prize for physics, has long argued that human 'quality' is declining, for which, he argues, we need corrective measures. Part of the correction is to ensure the breeding of 'high quality' people – such as winners of the Nobel Prize. For this reason, Shockley has contributed to a sperm bank set up for the sperm of 'superintelligent' men. When he contributed to this, Shockley had already fathered three children: Gena Corea, in her book *The Mother Machine* asks:

> Did Shockley's own three children, engendered when he was younger, turn out to be brilliant, 'more ideal' human beings? Measured against himself, he judges, his children 'represent a very significant regression'. But that does not mean his sperm is faulty. The eggs were to blame: 'My first wife – their mother – had not as high an academic-achievement standing as I had.'[4]

Most scientists ridicule this extreme belief in the importance of the genes in determining offspring 'quality'.

As long as AID is in medical control, there is also a risk that women with infertility problems may be denied access to sperm banks because they are considered 'unsuitable'. Lesbians and single women may be denied access to AID through clinics because they are not part of a 'family', while women with disabilities might be denied access, in the belief that they 'should not' reproduce. This belief may partly have to do with attitudes that assume that people with disabilities are somehow incapable of sex and reproduction, and partly to do with fears about the inheritability of disabilities.

The attitude that disabled people somehow 'should not' reproduce is allied to a belief that it is immoral to knowingly conceive a child who might inherit a disabling disease (see also chapter 7). One American theologian, Joseph Fletcher, argued that, if we are concerned about child abuse, then we should also recognise that children are 'abused' prenatally:

> ... not only by their mothers drinking alcohol, smoking, and using drugs non-medicinally; but also by their *knowingly* passing on, or risking passing on, genetic diseases ... If reproductive partners are informed they both carry a dread disease such as Tay-Sachs or cystic fibrosis, yet even so conceive with the intention of bringing every conceptus to birth, their supposed right to reproduce becomes ethically invalid.[5]

Because some kinds of disability are undoubtedly genetic, there is a danger that the medical profession will generalise to all women with any kind of disability, inheritable or not, and deny them access to infertility services, including one of the most simple, AID.

Fertilisation through self-insemination (SI) at home is one way for women to avoid medical control. Some women may choose to do this, using donated sperm, if they have experienced fertility problems resulting from their partner's low sperm count. But many women using SI have had no fertility problems, rather, they are often women who want to conceive without sexual contact with men. Confronted with the power of medicine, feminist self-help health groups have found many ways of taking control into their own hands. Feminist self-insemination groups are one way of doing so.

These are groups of women who meet together partly to talk about self-insemination and its implications for women, and also to organise it for themselves.[6]

These women may see SI, as the Feminist Self-Insemination Group have pointed out, as more than the mere act of getting pregnant without heterosexual intercourse. Rather,

> It is nothing less than a radically different approach to the concept of biological parenting as well as to the question of 'what *kind* of children do I want?'. SI has decisive implications on the concept of biological parenting – of who the sperm donors are and who will be the future 'family' of the child, including the biological and non-biological mother(s) and friends of both sexes.[7]

Self-insemination, then, doesn't avoid altogether the issue of quality control. What it does do is to put that 'quality control' back in the hands of the women who want to bear children. To put control back into women's – rather than medical – hands is important, although it does not altogether avoid the issues raised by the selection of donors.

While traditionalists and lawyers are arguing over who is the 'real' father of a child born as a result of AID, many feminists involved in SI are busy raising children without a 'social' father present at all. Many of them have, moreover, used sperm from donors that many traditionalists would consider quite unsuitable as genetic fathers – gay men, for instance. Self-insemination does allow women to challenge traditional notions of the family. And, because it is not a highly technological kind of intervention, it allows them to do so without medical control. That is not the case, however, with fertilisation taking place outside a woman's body, as in IVF.

In Vitro Fertilisation: Creating Embryos in the Lab

The treatment of infertility has traditionally had a low priority in the health services. Partly, this has to do with the more widespread problem of resources within an increasingly stretched NHS. It also has to do with the attitudes of gynaecologists towards infertility. As Naomi Pfeffer has pointed out,

> the medical management of infertility has been unpopular with gynaecologists not only because of its intimate and sordid nature but because prior to the introduction of in vitro fertilisation and embryo transfer, those treating infertility could make few claims to special knowledge and treatment.[8]

Techniques such as IVF have changed that (see box 5.4). There is no doubt that the introduction of technology has altered the status of practitioners. There is equally little doubt that women undergoing IVF do not have much control over the procedure. The most difficult part of IVF is obtaining eggs for possible fertilisation outside the woman's body. This requires hormones, and methods to 'see' her ovaries, and to obtain any eggs. None of these are straightforward procedures, and all can cause a woman pain and/or discomfort. The hormone treatments, as we have seen, may provoke nausea or abdominal discomfort; ultrasound imaging may be uncomfortable or even painful when it is used to visualise the ovaries through the woman's abdominal wall (this is usually done only when the bladder is full). Some methods of obtaining eggs, and the procedures involved in the final replacement of any embryos, may involve general anaesthesia, not necessarily painful, but a procedure that certainly carries some risk.

Yet it is not, primarily, these risks that have invoked controversy either from traditionalist or feminist perspectives. Most critics are alarmed by techniques such as IVF, because it seems to involve intensive medical intervention into an area of life that somehow seems sacrosanct. The opposition centres on the fact that fertilisation – the creation of an early embryo – occurs outside the body. It is not just that a third party, and technology, is involved: what is also important is the method of fertilisation itself. Thus, SPUC are

Box 5.4. *What is In Vitro Fertilisation?*

IVF means fertilisation in glass (in vitro) – i.e. in the laboratory dish. Although it is hailed as a breakthrough, many of the techniques it employs have been available for some time. Scientists in the nineteenth century discovered that animal cells could be kept alive and made to divide (this is called culturing them) in laboratory dishes, provided they put the cells into special nutrient solutions. And laparoscopy – the technique used by doctors to look at the woman's internal organs through a kind of telescope – was invented in the early years of this century.

An important step in developing the techniques was the discovery, in the 1950s and 1960s, that hormones from the pituitary can be used to overcome some kinds of infertility, by stimulating ovaries to produce mature eggs. This is still the first step involved in retrieving eggs for IVF (see box 4.3). In most cases, the timing of the last hormone injection allows doctors to predict when the hormone surge will occur that results in ovulation. They will then retrieve eggs through a tube that has been passed through the woman's abdomen (or, in newer techniques, through her vagina and bladder) and transfer them to a culture solution. This has been prepared in advance, using blood serum obtained from the woman herself.

Meanwhile, the man's sperm are obtained about thirty minutes before the doctors remove the woman's eggs. But the sperm cannot just be placed into the dish with the egg. They, too, have to be specially prepared: one essential step is that they have to be removed from the surrounding liquid (semen), as this contains something that inhibits their fertilising capacity. Then the prepared egg(s) are transferred to the dish containing the prepared sperm, and left for another twenty-four hours. After this, scientists inspect the dishes for evidence of early development: if this is happening, the embryo(s) will have to be transferred into the woman's body. This is usually done with the woman under general anaesthesia; the doctor

(*Continued overleaf*)

> puts a fine tube through the woman's cervix, and into her uterus, expelling the embryos high into the cavity.
>
> Some doctors prefer to freeze the embryos immediately after fertilisation, and then to transfer them to the woman in her next menstrual cycle. The reason for this is that the rather high levels of hormones used to make the woman produce more eggs than usual, so that they can be retrieved, tends to reduce the chances of pregnancy: probably, the hormones do something to make the woman's uterus less able to accept any embryo. So, freezing the embryo and waiting until the next cycle is one way of avoiding this problem.

less critical of techniques that involve removing eggs from a woman's body, if those eggs are then replaced into her body for fertilisation by 'sperm . . . already supplied by normal intercourse',[9] than they are of IVF itself where fertilisation takes place in the laboratory.[10]

The reason for this distinction has to do with arguments about the moral status of human embryos. Because embryos have the potential to become humans, the argument goes, they should be accorded human rights. This, not surprisingly, is the argument put forward by anti-abortion agencies, who claim that abortion, however early in gestation, constitutes murder of a potential, or actual, human life.

According to this view, the 'loss' of any of these eggs or embryos, *even before implantation*, constitutes a death. Thus, SPUC claim, for instance, that the chances of becoming pregnant with one fetus are only 40 per cent even after the transfer of three embryos (in IVF) for three cycles, that is, to a total of nine transferred embryos. They argue that 'to offer an infertile woman a 40 per cent chance of achieving implantation . . . the loss of up to eight sibling embryos has to be an acceptable prospect'.[11] In other words, even if a woman is one of the 40 per cent who do become pregnant, eight more of her embryos have 'died'. That the embryo before implantation is a human 'baby', fully deserving of special protection, was echoed by one American doctor involved in the anti-abortion crusade, who railed against women's destruction of the

> ... children nestling within them – children fully alive from the moment of conception [i.e. fertilisation] that have already been fully detached from all organic connection with their parent [i.e. as the fertilised egg moves along the Fallopian tube prior to implantation] and only re-attached to her for the purpose of nutriment and growth.[12]

There has, however, been feminist opposition to the claim of moral status for fetuses. Such opposition rests on the claim that any rights to which a fetus might be due should not outweigh the rights of the woman who carries it. Feminist organisations have, through various campaigns, consistently maintained women's rights to abortion facilities. Although opponents of abortion have claimed that feminists therefore have no regard for the fetus, the demand for women's rights to abortion has not claimed that fetuses have no rights, nor that we have no duty to protect them.

In this way, feminists challenge the claim that a fetus has the same moral status as a child or an adult. It does not challenge another assumption underpinning the traditionalist view; that is, the assertion that there is a biological and moral continuity between the fertilised egg and the newborn baby.

What is significant about the claim for moral status of the early human embryo in debates about IVF is precisely that the woman's body is ignored. 'Capacity to become human' thus resides only in the genetic information possessed by a dividing fertilised egg. Yet, as we have seen earlier, that capacity to become human is not realisable unless that egg becomes implanted into a woman's uterus. Human potentiality is, in short, realised only when the embryo is in intimate interaction with a woman's biology. And even then it remains only a relative possibility: all kinds of problems may yet occur which obliterate that potential. An early fetus that miscarries, for instance, inevitably fails to realise its 'human' potential.

At the stage when eggs that have been fertilised in vitro are ready to be put back into a woman, they have begun to divide. By fourteen days (the maximum period permitted under Warnock recommendations), the 'embryo' has few features; it is just beginning to develop the 'primitive streak', the first real sign that any structures are emerging from what is, till then, merely a ball of cells. It is just because of this lack of differentiation at such early stages that some doctors prefer to refer to a 'pre-embryo'. Even at this stage, there is no way of knowing which cells are going to form which bits, which cells are going to become the fetus, or even whether any are going to form a fetus at all (see box 5.5). As we have seen, it is simply not biologically correct to assume that potential humans unfold from the dividing cells of the newly fertilised egg.

An important problem for feminists with the idea of unfolding from a blueprint written into our genes is that it treats the embryo (or later, the fetus) as though it has no environment, no context. Ros Petchesky has described[13] how photographic images of fetuses as somehow floating freely in fluid-filled space has helped to create an ideology of fetuses as morally alone – as alone as the individual adult that they will one day become. They are also portrayed as competent, doing things that older babies will do (sucking a thumb, for example). The embryo has only to grow and break out of its watery world; so, a fetus with its thumb in its mouth is seen to be morally *the same as* a baby that sucks its thumb. But in practice, an embryo has actively to *become*, or be made into, a fetus, and whatever fetuses do in the uterus is not at all the same as what they would do after birth.

Does such biological detail matter to feminism? Feminists have voiced concern about IVF and associated technologies on various grounds; but feminists have said rather little about the fate of any pre-embryos that are not put back into the

> **Box 5.5. *Blueprints for Babies?***
>
> What genes do is sometimes, erroneously, described in terms of a 'blueprint', a 'plan for the organism', rather like a plan for a house. All that is then required to make an animal, say, is to 'read' the plans and assemble the building materials into the planned shape. But how different shapes (of animals or plants) arise in nature is one of the biggest problems in science. Biologists cannot yet explain how shapes arise or how they change during development. Information in genes certainly does not explain biological form – how, for instance, does the *same* set of genes determine the transition between the very different shapes of a tadpole and an adult frog? All that we know about genes is that they determine the order in which 'building blocks' are assembled to make a particular protein. We don't even know how the complex three-dimensional shape of the protein is determined. However they work, the information contained in its genes may (or may not) be used by the organism itself as it develops – quite unlike a 'developing' building which does not.

woman's womb, but are kept for research. We have, rather, been forced into arguing that embryos don't much matter, in order to safeguard women's right to choose abortion. Yet we do have to recognise that not all women will react to images of 'unwanted embryos' being thrown down the sink with indifference. Ros Petchesky, in her analysis of the role of 'fetal images', points out how cultural representations help to determine the meaning of pregnancy for women: because those cultural images specifically include the portrayal of fetuses as lone travellers, some women may see in discarded pre-embryos an identification with a potential baby.

The imagery employed in media representations of IVF certainly encourages women (and men) to see pre-embryos as potential people. Photographs of the cluster of eight or sixteen cells that is to be transferred to the waiting woman's womb sit alongside photographs of smiling mothers and babies, or of the inevitable lone fetus, sucking its thumb. Women are encouraged to look down the microscope to see 'their' embryos prior to replacement. Just as seeing ultrasound images of 'their baby' during pregnancy helps to 'make the baby more real' for women, so seeing what has happened since fertilisation helps women to identify with that ball of cells. In the process, it becomes synonymous with 'my baby'.

That process is not possible with the newer techniques that involve fertilisation inside a woman's body, using eggs that doctors have extracted in a similar way to IVF. GIFT (Gamete Intra-Fallopian Transfer) entails extracting eggs, using the techniques we have already outlined for IVF, and mixing them with sperm in the laboratory. But, rather than then waiting for fertilisation to take place in vitro, the mixed eggs and sperm are transferred immediately to the woman's Fallopian tube.

GIFT is used by some clinics as an alternative to IVF. Doctors see it as a useful alternative for couples with 'unexplained infertility', or for anyone who has religious or moral reasons to oppose fertilisation outside the body. If more eggs are removed than are replaced (usually two eggs per tube), then the remainder can be fertilised and frozen in case fertilisation through GIFT fails. If it does, then the doctor may suggest in vitro fertilisation at the appropriate time in the next cycle.

A newer version is called POST (Peritoneal Ovum-Sperm Transfer; see box 5.6), in which the eggs and sperm are transferred into a part of the abdominal cavity, just behind the woman's womb. This space, the Pouch of Douglas, is relatively easy to locate, so laparoscopy (using a fine 'telescope' to locate specific parts of the reproductive tract) isn't necessary. One important consequence of that is that it can be done under local, rather than general, anaesthesia.

One objection to IVF raised by some feminist critics is that, despite massive and risky interventions, it has a very low success rate, leading at best to 9 per cent successes (measured

Box 5.6. *Some Techniques Used With IVF, and Their Names*

You will come across a variety of techniques, all with different names, in newspaper reports of IVF. These are changing all the time, but the general principles remain roughly the same.

First of all, there are two stages to all techniques: (i) obtaining gametes; that is, eggs and sperm; and (ii) fertilisation. If fertilisation takes place *outside* the body, there is a third stage, (iii) putting the product of fertilisation back into the woman's body.

The various techniques differ in: (a) how eggs are removed; (b) what is put back into the woman's body; (c) where they are put back; and (d) how they are put back.

(a) Eggs may be removed by laparoscopy through the woman's abdominal wall. Doctors use an ultrasound scan over her abdomen to locate her ovaries, and obtains the eggs through a needle passed through her abdomen. This method can be painful because this kind of ultrasound requires a full bladder. Alternatively, a newer kind of ultrasound device uses a vaginal probe, to which the egg-collecting needle is attached. This does not need a full bladder to visualise the ovaries.

(b) What is put back into a woman's body may be an early, developing embryo (embryo transfer) following fertilisation in vitro. Or, doctors may transfer the zygote (the fertilised egg, before it begins development) or the gametes (eggs and sperm) themselves.

(c) Where it is put back depends upon what is transferred. If it has begun to develop (as in embryo transfer), the embryo is usually transferred to the uterus, because that is where it would have got to if it had been fertilised normally and travelled along the Fallopian tube. This procedure is necessary in women whose infertility results from blocked tubes. In the case of zygotes, or gametes, they may be transferred directly to the Fallopian tubes (as in GIFT) because that is where fertilisation would normally take place. Sometimes gametes are transferred into the woman's abdomen, as in POST.

(d) If embryos are transferred directly into the uterus, they

(*Continued overleaf*)

> can be inserted directly via the vagina. But if gametes or zygotes are transferred into specific locations further inside the body (such as the Fallopian tubes) they have to be transferred using laparoscopy and ultrasound.
>
> How doctors decide which method to use depends upon cost, the medical reasons for a particular woman's infertility treatment, and the risks attached to certain procedures.

as numbers of live babies born per attempt at retrieving eggs, calculated for US clinics in 1986[14]). This is perhaps not a particularly useful criticism: some of the risks associated with these procedures (e.g. anaesthesia) are reduced by techniques like POST, and the success rate of these techniques taken together is increasing (e.g. in one study of women undergoing GIFT, 40 per cent of women whose eggs had been replaced into both Fallopian tubes became pregnant, compared to initial pregnancy rates of 14 per cent for IVF: the percentage of babies born is, of course, less for both procedures.)[15] The success rate may well improve when more is known about different pre-embryos: a number of research teams have found chemical differences between 'good' pre-embryos (i.e. those that are likely to become implanted in the woman's womb) and 'bad' ones (those that are not likely to do so). Those differences could become the basis for chemical testing of pre-embryos in IVF procedures, so ensuring a better success rate[16] (although there will inevitably be a limit to potential success rates: not all embryos that are fertilised naturally will implant, after all).

Criticising the success or failure of the technology in its own terms may not be a useful strategy for feminists for just these reasons: successes are limited partly by the 'natural' processes over which scientists currently have no control (implantation, for example), and scientific 'progress' will inevitably bring refinements of the technology. What is important is whether it will ever become cost-effective. At the moment, not only are the techniques not particularly successful, but they are also rather costly; and, not surprisingly, they are quite difficult to obtain within the NHS.

What about other criticisms feminists have of techniques such as IVF? Perhaps the strongest claim is that the technology enhances men's ability to control female reproduction directly, thus enhancing patriarchal control of women. There is no doubt that IVF involves considerable technical intervention, and that this can be seen against a backdrop of increased medical intervention in reproduction. The 'medical management' of labour has been with us for thirty years.

Still, there are problems with this claim. In the first place, it invokes an image of a slippery slope towards the eventual production of babies completely in the laboratory. Women would then become redundant, they argue, or reduced to the level of egg-machines. This is to define women in terms of our role in biological reproduction (a dangerous definition), and also portrays patriarchy as inevitably the same in the future. What remains unclear in these analyses is how a future patriarchy would fund such a costly exercise, and why it should want to do so: women are, after all, likely to be cheaper. This pessimistic vision in turn defines women as passive victims, unable to resist the increasing control of that universal patriarchy. Yet, as several feminist writers have pointed out, women do resist and have generated demands for particular technologies (e.g. epidural anaesthesia in childbirth) as well as resisting others (e.g. over-enthusiastic use of fetal monitoring).

Referring to the control over women by men may be overgeneralising. There is no doubt that the gynaecologist carrying out the procedures is in a powerful position with respect to the infertile woman: not only is that potentially true of any doctor–patient relationship, but he (for it usually is he in IVF clinics) has the skills that might enable the woman to achieve the desired pregnancy. But we should remember that the gynaecologist is *also* in a powerful position in relation to the woman's male partner. The partner may know that his sperm count is normal: but the fact remains that he has not succeeded in impregnating his wife/lover. Indeed, it is no accident that media portrayals of 'miracle babies' following IVF often refer to the gynaecologist as though he is the 'father' of the child – and rarely show pictures of the infertile father with the bouncing baby. Even though he undoubtedly gains some benefit from the intervention, the male partner becomes invisible.

Women could resist the apparent increase in 'technological management', epitomised by IVF, but, on the whole, have not. We have tended to remain ambivalent. On the one hand, we have tended to recognise that women, for various reasons, might want to have children, and that should be a woman's choice. If so, then it should be like abortion: freely available to all women, and as safe as medical technology and know-how will allow. That is, as with abortion, we should not oppose the technology itself, but rather should voice our opposition to the ways in which it is organised[17].

On the other hand, despite media images of science as progress, most women are distrustful of, and alienated from, scientific knowledge. It is, then, not surprising that some feminist writers have emphasised the slippery slope towards a world in which more and more aspects of pregnancy are taken outside of our bodies, until bearing children might be removed from women's bodies entirely, and into the hands of (male) scientists. But in practice, even if that is the long-term goal of some scientists working in this field, the trend at present is towards making *fewer*, not more, interventions outside the body; the newer technique of GIFT, for instance, requires extracting eggs, but then allowing fertilisation to occur inside the woman's body. Whatever the ultimate motivation of individuals, the research is inevitably limited by cost. GIFT is slightly cheaper than IVF simply because much less is done outside the body, and no special solutions are required to maintain the fertilised eggs.

Cost is the main factor limiting the extent of technological intervention in pregnancy. Most IVF clinics are private, so the entire costs of the procedure (in staffing, general overheads, equipment, and so on) are borne by the patients. Of those offering IVF within the NHS, nearly all operate a mixture of NHS and private practice. A clinic in Oxford, for instance, charges patients only for the actual cost of treatment (£750 per cycle), while all the hospital backup is met out of NHS budgets. King's College Hospital operates a 'support group', which is a registered charity and raises funds towards the running costs of the IVF programme.

That NHS resources are used to back up provision for private patients is not new; however, in relation to IVF programmes, there is a difference. Unlike many cases requiring costly forms of hospital treatment, women undergoing IVF are not actually ill: infertility may be traumatic and difficult to live with, but it is not life-threatening. Moreover, the depletion of NHS resources means that less money is available to fund research into other methods of treating infertility, or into the causes of infertility – many of which may be easily preventable.

That the success rate of IVF in enabling infertile women to achieve pregnancy is low, while the treatment is expensive, has been one of the major planks of feminist criticism. Critics have pointed out that the statistics given are often misleading, or are reported inaccurately in media reports. One reason why they are misleading is that clinical reports typically refer, say, to the rate of clinical pregnancies per embryo transfer. But embryo transfer is the final step in a series of procedures – and for the woman, clinical pregnancy may not mean a baby. This kind of calculation ignores the number of women who fail to respond to hormone treatments, who drop out of the programme, whose eggs are not fertilised, or who lose their pregnancies. As one medical report put it, '. . . the most relevant figure for a patient is the so-called take-home baby rate' – the percentage of live births for each step of the process. That rate is, as critics have underlined, quite dismal. Only about 7 per cent of all hormonally stimulated menstrual cycles lead to the birth of a live baby, while 9 per cent of egg retrievals lead to a birth, and 11 per cent of embryo transfers[18]. Still, the newer developments, such as GIFT and POST may turn out to be both more successful in terms of babies born, and less expensive. Even so, it is unlikely that they will be available freely to all women. Thus, if we accept the techniques – or at least their inevitability – then we must campaign to increase their availability.

But what of the stronger feminist criticisms? Some feminists react to the technology of IVF with revulsion, particularly at the degree of male medical control over women's bodies. There is no doubt that IVF represents control, but just how different is it from other medical (or non-medical) procedures? The final stage of IVF itself is the introduction of the embryo or embryos into the woman's uterus. This procedure is usually done through her vagina, so that the doctor inserts the embryos through her cervix. This is, in effect, little different from artificial insemination, when it is carried out in a medical context. So this stage, at least, is no more, or less, controlling than other techniques.

What makes IVF both excitingly new (for media representations) and more threatening (for many feminists) is the way that all these various components have been brought together. Each one on their own is costly, and the combination is more expensive still. Each requires medical skill, but the combination requires considerable expertise, especially in the surgical procedures involved in extracting the prepared eggs. That ability to bring different components of medical procedure together may, in the future, enable scientists or doctors to control other aspects of pregnancy. At present, 'high technology' is involved mainly in the very first steps, harvesting eggs, bringing them together with sperm, and maintaining embryos in solution or in the deep freeze: highly technological interventions have not yet intervened in later stages of pregnancy (although 'fetal surgery' is a growing specialism). Implantation and early pregnancy raise many other issues (including prenatal diagnoses, and selective abortions, discussed in Chapter Seven), but, in themselves, they are not presently subject to much technical control. If scientists know rather little about the mechanics of fertilisation, they know even less about how early embryos manage to implant into the womb.

6. What Can Go Wrong? Implantation and Pregnancy

After fertilisation the possibilities for technological intervention are rather more limited. Whatever the fears of many critics of reproductive technology that we are on a slippery path towards a technological takeover, with the production of babies taking place entirely in the laboratory, the fact is that scientists currently know far too little to be able to exert extensive control over biological events of early pregnancy.

The next stage after fertilisation is implantation, the process in which the embryo becomes attached to the womb. But despite its fascination for scientists, they know too little about the mechanisms of implantation to be able to intervene in it to any great extent. Indeed, it is just that lack of knowledge that represents the major *failure* of IVF – although media reports rarely acknowledge it. However good a particular doctor is at extracting eggs and replacing them after fertilisation, implantation itself may fail, often for inexplicable reasons. In short, the success or failure of the technique depends on what happens next: and what happens next depends crucially on the mother, as well as on the embryo.

For many women, failing to have babies has little to do with their ability to produce eggs, or to do with their male partner's sperm. For some unknown reasons, such women either do not manage to retain a fertilised egg long enough for it to implant, or, if it implants, it does not stay there. When that happens, most people call it a miscarriage, while doctors refer to it as a spontaneous abortion. As many as seven out of ten conceptions are estimated either to fail to implant or to miscarry early in pregnancy. If miscarriage occurs after implantation, then the woman will usually know that she has been pregnant: the miscarriage will show as heavy bleeding. Most women find miscarriage a traumatic and unhappy experience, giving them a sense of loss. One woman commented:

> The miscarriage was also a bereavement, in the real sense of the word. I'm approaching the time when it would have been due, and as that gets closer, I get more and more sad and depressed about it.[1]

But if the miscarriage occurred before, or even in the few days immediately after, implantation a woman would be unlikely to know that she had conceived: all that she might notice is a heavier-than-usual period. Because the woman would not know that she had been pregnant, it is hard to estimate how many human eggs are conceived but subsequently lost. Still, doctors have estimated that the probability of producing a baby following unprotected intercourse at the time of ovulation is only about 25 per cent (in the other 75 per cent of cases, either no fertilisation occurs or the embryo subsequently fails). And even of those embryos that do succeed in implanting, 50 per cent of them will subsequently die long before birth.

There are several reasons why this high rate of loss of early embryos occurs. One is simply that the woman's uterus is not in a sufficiently 'prepared' state for the embryo to attach (see box 6.1); this could be due to hormonal imbalance, or because there is something clinically wrong, such as a cervix that is slightly open (called 'incompetent cervix'), or fibroids in the uterus. In cases like these, a doctor may recommend surgery (to correct the opening of the cervix, for example). If a hormone imbalance is the cause of repeated miscarriages, then doctors may recommend hormone treatments. These are, however, controversial; not everyone is convinced that

Box 6.1. *Implantation 1: What do Embryos Have to Do?*

The processes involved in an embryo becoming implanted into the wall of the womb are complex and poorly understood. Scientists have only recently begun to recognise the intricacies of the interaction between the embryo and the uterus: some refer to it as a 'conversation', for which both participants must be ready. Putting an embryo into a womb unprepared for it will not lead to pregnancy.

By the time it enters the uterus, the fertilised egg has divided to become a ball of cells called the blastocyst. On its way, this ball secretes a hormone that affects the woman's ovaries, in turn making them secrete another hormone (progesterone) that is essential to prepare the uterus. As the ball approaches the wall of the uterus, two things have to happen. First, it 'hatches' from its outermost coat, the zona, and secondly, it has to attach itself to the uterine wall. 'Hatching' from the zona is sometimes harder for the embryo to achieve after in vitro fertilisation (for unknown reasons).

As it approaches the wall of the uterus, electrical and chemical changes occur in both the pre-embryo (a rather arbitrary term for embryos in the first fourteen days) and the adjacent wall: no one knows how these changes are synchronised. Once it has met up with the wall, a chemical change occurs that spreads rapidly throughout the muscle of the uterus, which helps to prepare it for implantation (see box 6.2).

Once a human embryo has attached to the wall, it literally eats its way in, digesting that part of the wall as it does so and using the digested material to 'feed' the growing embryo. Within a few days (between seven and twelve days after fertilisation) it has become incorporated *into* the wall, even eating into some of the mother's blood vessels so that the outer layer of the embryo (that will eventually become its 'coat' of membranes and the placenta) is bathed in maternal blood.

Box 6.2. *Implantation 2: The Role of the Uterus*

As the embryo enters it, the uterus has already become prepared for it by the hormones secreted from the ovaries. These help to build up a thick and secretory lining (which comes away as menstruation if no implantation occurs). As soon as the embryo becomes attached, chemical changes occur, although scientists have not yet identified exactly what causes these rapid changes in the uterine wall. None of these changes is possible if the balance of hormones is not right: if, for instance, the embryo does not stimulate the ovaries with enough of *its* hormone, the uterine wall cannot respond adequately. If that happens, the embryo will die and be washed out as the uterine walls break down at menstruation.

These changes in the uterus do several things. First, they help to promote the growth of tiny blood vessels (capillaries) just beneath the embryo as it attaches to the uterus: eventually, these will form part of the placenta that will provide the growing fetus with nourishment. Second, the uterus begins to secrete various chemicals which probably help to control the environment of the embryo: one chemical, for instance, might help to regulate water balance around the embryo before the placenta itself has fully formed. Third, changes in the uterus may help to protect the embryo from the woman's immune system. The embryo is genetically different from its mother: if tissues that are genetically different are transplanted surgically into people, their bodies would recognise the difference and reject the grafted tissue (surgeons try to avoid this in organ transplants by suppressing the patient's immune system with drugs). But most fetuses are not rejected. Scientists do not know why in detail, although it seems that the invading embryo secretes hormones that moderate the mother's immune system.

Another result of these changes in the uterus is that the uterus itself is protected from too much damage by the invading embryo. If the changes are not adequate, then the

(Continued overleaf)

> embryo may invade too deeply, causing damage. Embryos are also more invasive when they land up in other places outside the uterus, where these changes do not normally take place (such as the wall of the gut). This happens, for instance, in ectopic pregnancy.

there is sufficient evidence that hormone treatment helps, and, as we have seen, giving hormones in early pregnancy *may* pose risks to the fetus.

Another reason is when the embryo begins to attach and the mother's immune system begins to reject it (see box 6.2). For some unknown reason fetuses are more likely to be rejected by the mother's body if they are chemically similar in certain ways to her, which may occur if she is very similar, chemically, to her partner (this is quite unlike the way that immune systems work normally). This probably explains why miscarriages are more common among very inbred groups of people. Some doctors have tried immunising women against their partners' sperm, so that their bodies recognise the fetus as different; but this is still experimental.

Perhaps the major reason why early embryos abort is that something is genetically wrong with them, such as having the 'wrong' number of chromosomes (see box 6.3). Unlike physical problems, which can sometimes be corrected surgically to prevent repeated miscarriage, there is little that can be done about abortion due to genetic defect. But on the other hand, it is rarely a cause of *repeated* miscarriage, unless, say, both parents pass on a severe chromosomal abnormality. Both parents could have such an abnormality in a form that has never showed up in their own lives, but does every time the woman's eggs are fertilised creating an embryo having two such abnormal chromosomes. If the abnormality is particularly severe, all fetuses inheriting those chromosomes will die. Still, the chances of that are quite small. The vast majority of miscarriages occur because, by chance, something has gone genetically wrong with the development of *that particular* embryo (see Chapter Seven); the miscarriage is then an isolated event, unlikely to be repeated in subsequent pregnancies.

That so many early embryos fail to establish a pregnancy following 'natural' intercourse needs to be weighed against the claim that in vitro fertilisation is not particularly successful. IVF, after all, is likely to be used to treat women who are somewhat older than the average age of women who conceive naturally: most are in their mid to late thirties by the time they enter treatment. At that age, the rates of 'natural' conception are beginning to decline. Whether fertilisation occurs inside or outside a woman's body, the chances that her uterus will accept an implanting embryo decline sharply after she is about forty years old. Even so, estimates of the number of women whose embryos do implant after fertilisation in vitro suggest that, in some clinics, between 20 and 35 per cent of women who had never previously been pregnant have had embryos implant.

However the success rate of IVF is assessed (and its assessment is controversial), the technical problems that it presents arise mainly from the lack of control that scientists can exert after the embryos have been transferred. Provided that a woman's ovaries respond to the 'shots' of hormones by producing mature eggs, and that her partner produces 'normal' sperm, then that part of the process is relatively controllable; so there is a reasonable chance that fertilisation itself can take place. It is after the embryos are put back, and events are 'in nature's hands' that many of the problems attributed to IVF are likely to occur, simply because no one can predict with any accuracy quite how a woman's body is going to respond. As Ann Oakley has commented,

> ... if women are to bear healthy babies and retain their own health in the process ... it is not sufficient to trust Nature – significantly dubbed *Mother* Nature precisely for her unreliability in this regard? Natural processes are wasteful of human life

> **Box 6.3. Why Do Embryos Abort? Extra Chromosomes and Down's Syndrome**
>
> Human cells, including cells of human embryos, normally contain twenty-three pairs of chromosomes – forty-six in all. Sometimes, though, embryos begin to develop that contain forty-seven rather than forty-six. Usually, the extra chromosome gets there because the egg did not develop properly in its early stages: to make forty-six *after* fertilisation, eggs and sperm have to divide in a special way so that their pairs of chromosomes are split, and each egg or sperm gets one of each pair (twenty-three altogether). But occasionally, this splitting does not happen to all the pairs, and so an egg or sperm is formed with twenty-four chromosomes. This happens more often to eggs, because they undergo the first part of their development around the time of the woman's *own* birth – and so wait many years before they have to undergo the rest of their development. So, acquiring 'extra' chromosomes is more likely when the woman is older than forty.
>
> The best known example of 'extra' chromosomes is Down's syndrome (babies born with an extra chromosome number twenty-one). Embryos that have an extra one of most of the other chromosomes, however, are likely to be highly abnormal and to abort very early in pregnancy. We don't know if many embryos form that have one too few chromosomes. The only one that ever survives is one having a sex chromosome missing. No others have ever been found. Since it is theoretically possible for them to occur, their absence is probably because they are so grossly abnormal that they do not even get to the stage of implantation.

and humans have invented the resources to do something about this wastefulness.[2]

Nature's wastefulness has not, perhaps, been at the forefront of feminist concern about IVF. But what does provoke questions is medical attempts to 'do something' about that wastefulness in early pregnancy. One avenue of control is through embryo transfer, the final stage of the IVF process. By transferring only those embryos they identify as viable doctors aim to reduce that 'wastefulness'.

The Fate of Embryos After IVF; Embryo Transfer

Embryos produced through IVF face one of several futures. Some of them will be replaced into a woman's body, perhaps to begin development as a fetus. Others may be frozen, for possible transfer to a woman's body at some later date. In principle, yet others could either be thrown away, or used in research. All of these fates have aroused controversy.

Embryo transfer (ET) certainly raises several issues for feminists. ET (see box 6.4) is one part of IVF; once the egg has been fertilised in the laboratory, the embryo is usually allowed to develop until it consists of a ball of eight or sixteen cells. At this stage, it is transferred back into the woman's body. This is normally the woman from whom the eggs were extracted; but ET has also been carried out with eggs donated by another woman. Egg donation has, like sperm donation, been somewhat controversial; for feminists, it raises many of the same questions as surrogacy.

One criticism of IVF is that it leads to a greater number of abnormal pregnancies than does 'normal' fertilisation. Ectopic pregnancies (occurring outside the womb, e.g. in the Fallopian tubes, or in the abdomen) are more common following IVF, and pose considerable danger to the woman's health and life. No one really knows why such problems are more likely; nor do they know whether the problems arise because fertilisation occurs outside the body, and are connected with the process of transferring embryos, or are caused by the original reasons for the infertility. Just because ET is, at present, rarely practised in humans *without* the techniques of IVF, it is virtually impossible to tease these apart.

Certainly some of the things that can go 'wrong' with early

Box 6.4. *What is Embryo Transfer?*

Embryo transfer (ET) is, quite simply, the process of taking embryos that have been cultured in the laboratory and replacing them into a female body for (possible) implantation. There are, in principle, two ways in which scientists obtain embryos. First, they could obtain eggs and sperm, and then allow fertilisation to occur in the lab: this is the basis of IVF. Second, they could obtain embryos from inside the female reproductive system after fertilisation has occurred there. To do this, the scientists have to 'wash out' the embryos, a technique called embryo flushing. Embryo flushing is used fairly commonly in agriculture, as it is less expensive (and less traumatic for the animal) than obtaining eggs by laparoscopy. A few doctors have used this technique with women, but its practice is still rare.

Agricultural scientists are developing a system of animal breeding called MOET (multiple ovulation and embryo transfer). First, they give a donor cow or ewe hormones to make her produce multiple eggs, and then inseminate her artificially. After that, any resulting embryos are flushed out, for transfer to other (usually less valuable) 'carrier' females. This system is too expensive to be used commercially on any large scale simply to produce high quality animals in larger numbers (although it is used more extensively in the US than in Europe). But it does enable scientists to increase dramatically the speed with which genetic improvements can be made in breeding stock (until the new technologies were developed, agriculture relied on selective breeding of animals of specified pedigrees).

Whether in agriculture or in medicine, embryos are usually transferred into a female recipient through her cervix. The embryos are flushed into a fine tube passing through her cervix and into her uterus. Some doctors may give a woman hormones at the time she has ET, in the belief that the compounds (e.g. progesterone) will help to 'boost' her own hormones: progesterone is the hormone that is normally produced by a woman's ovaries after ovulation, and helps to

> prepare her womb for implantation. The most controversial aspect of ET is that it allows embryos to be transferred into the womb of a woman even if the embryos are not 'hers' (i.e. from her eggs).

pregnancy following IVF and ET may be attributable to the techniques involved in maintaining and fertilising the eggs in the laboratory. The risk of identical twins (perhaps not a problem of pregnancy, although it may present problems for some parents) is thought to be greater with IVF. Identical twins arise because the fertilised egg divides into two separate halves before developing into genetically identical embryos. Some clinics have reported relatively high incidences of identical twin embryos after IVF and ET. The reasons are not known, although some scientists have suggested that it may have something to do with the way that the embryos are cultured in the laboratory (see box 6.1). Why this should result in twins is still a mystery, however.

Multiple pregnancies (i.e. two or more embryos implanted) are certainly more common in IVF and related procedures. One important reason for this is that the hormone treatments that are used are deliberately scaled so that *multiple* ovulation occurs. Having several eggs to fertilise allows doctors to transfer more than one embryo, so that there is a greater chance that at least one embryo will implant. As we have seen in Chapter Four, deciding how many embryos should be implanted has been a controversial question, with one clinic coming under fire because doctors there were transferring all embryos fertilised in vitro. Critics said that the risks of multiple pregnancy made this practice unethical. But, the clinic doctors argued, such multiple transfer was carried out only for women whose ovaries were polycystic (i.e. they had several ovarian cysts). Women with this condition had low chances of implanting an embryo anyway, so transferring large numbers of embryos increased their chances, the doctors believed.

The number of embryos transferred to a woman obviously affects how many embryos are likely to become implanted. But some doctors doing IVF work believe that numbers alone are not the only factor involved in creating multiple pregnancies. Evidence is scant, but it is possible, they believe, that as one transferred embryo begins to implant it 'helps' its sibs in some way. So, multiple pregnancies are also made more likely just because the first embryo has implanted successfully.

One reason why IVF and embryo transfer have acquired a name for low success rates is that, because of all the hormonal interference needed to get the eggs in the first place, the woman's cycle is altered. Her ovaries may respond to being over-stimulated by *failing* in their critical task of producing the hormone progesterone. And without that, her womb will not be in a state ready to maintain any embryo. Some doctors do advocate that women should be given injections of progesterone following IVF in an attempt to prevent this loss of pregnancy.

At the moment, no one knows whether exposing the migrating pre-embryo to such abnormal levels of hormones has deleterious effects on its development: all we know is that the rates of fetal abnormalities are not appreciably higher after in vitro fertilisation. Not surprisingly, attention has tended to focus on the extent to which these hormones mean risking the pregnancy itself. If there *is* any risk to the developing embryo, then that risk could be minimised if embryo transfer was postponed until the next cycle. This would mean that eggs would be extracted from a woman, and fertilised in vitro. But then, rather than transferring the resulting embryos, they would be frozen, and transferred to the woman only in the *next* cycle. Researchers have developed satisfactory ways of freezing embryos without damaging them only as recently as 1988; before that, embryos could be transferred only when freshly fertilised.

To some extent, keeping some embryos in reserve is practised already: any 'extra' embryos resulting from in vitro fertilisation may be saved and frozen, in preparation for the woman's next cycle should the first attempt fail. One advantage of postponing transfer may be that the transfer can then be done with only the woman's own hormones influencing the embryo: the disadvantage, though, is that too little is known about any potential hazards of freezing. Most thawed embryos do not appear to have suffered damage when they are inspected under a microscope, and healthy babies have been born after being frozen as embryos. But there may be slight risks that will come to light only when more such babies have been born. All we can say is that it *seems* safe at the moment.

Clinical discussions of the pros and cons of using hormones in conjunction with IVF programmes have centred on how well the hormones stimulate the ovaries to produce eggs. Much less obvious is any concern about deleterious effects of using such high levels of hormones. What is even less obvious is any reference in medical journals to the effects of these hormonal treatments – not on the developing embryo, or on the pregnancy, but on the woman. As one doctor explained, the drug clomiphene may make you 'feel a little unwell and very occasionally a few people [sic] get hot flushes when taking these pills. Since you are taking them for a limited time, these effects are hardly worth bothering about.'[3]

Still, women who want infertility treatment may well feel that they would put up with such 'bother' just for the chance to become pregnant. They might, on the other hand, be more concerned about possible effects of hormone treatment on the fetus. Early embryos at the time of implantation probably are not profoundly affected by hormones. Too much or too little of particular hormones at this time may affect the chances of implantation, but there is no clear evidence that they will affect the development of the early embryo once it has implanted. When hormones (and other chemicals) are most likely to affect a fetus is once its organs have begun to develop, around the fourth to twelfth weeks. Most IVF embryos/fetuses will be exposed only to the mother's hormones at that stage (just as will embryos conceived naturally). While it seems unlikely that IVF embryos are exposed to levels of hormones that might alter their development, doctors cannot yet be sure. We will know only when enough babies have been born through IVF.

Perhaps the greatest danger associated with IVF and embryo transfer is the risk of ectopic pregnancy. In Britain, about one pregnancy in 250 is ectopic (i.e. 0.4 per cent). These usually require surgery to remove the fetus, since there is a considerable risk that the fetus, growing in, for example, the Fallopian tube, may cause a rupture and life-threatening bleeding. There does seem to be a greater risk of ectopics after IVF and embryo transfer; estimates of rates vary from 2.3 per cent of pregnancies to 5 per cent. But what is less clear is why these techniques should be associated with greater risk of ectopics. In part, it may have something to do with the hormone treatment (there is a 3 per cent chance of ectopics following hormone treatment alone for infertility). It may also have something to do with the fact that women who have IVF are likely to have damaged tubes; this may contribute partly to the risk of ectopics because some of these women will have had previous surgery on the tubes in attempts to correct the damage – tubal surgery is known to increase the risk of ectopic pregnancy by nearly six times. Partly, too, infertility itself is associated with a risk, approximately three times greater than that of ectopic pregnancy.

Ectopic pregnancies are much rarer in populations of women in areas where pelvic inflammatory disease is unknown. PID is known to cause damage to the tubes – and hence contribute to infertility – and increases the risk of ectopics threefold. In pregnancies following normal fertilisation, ectopic pregnancy seems to be more likely with any condition (such as PID, use of an intra-uterine device, or treatment with hormones such as clomiphene) that slow down the passage of the fertilised egg through the Fallopian tube. Whether this is the case in ectopic pregnancies following IVF – or, indeed, whether they are associated with the IVF itself or the prior infertility – is unknown.

There is similar uncertainty about the reasons why spontaneous abortions are more likely following IVF and embryo transfer. The chances of miscarriage occurring increase as the woman gets older, which might be a factor – so might the various medical interventions used in obtaining eggs and replacing them after fertilisation. Some doctors involved in IVF, for instance, were initially afraid that there would be a higher than normal rate of embryos that tried to implant very low down in the uterus following replacement in the woman's body. If they did, they would be likely to abort. Whether this is a factor in the risk of miscarriage is unclear, although ultrasound scans to show the sites of implantation suggest otherwise.

Interpreting statistics about the successes or failures of IVF pregnancies is not easy. Women who have begun pregnancies conceived in vitro are much more likely to be monitored closely; they might, for instance, have ultrasound scans very early in pregnancy, to see how many embryos have implanted. Doing this has brought 'vanishing twins' to the attention of doctors: that is, an embryo that implants, but then becomes absorbed and disappears later in pregnancy, leaving its sibling to finish the pregnancy alone. This seems to be relatively common in pregnancies following IVF – but it does not happen *only* in IVF pregnancies. Until recently, doctors never offered ultrasound scans so early in pregnancy to women conceiving naturally. So, no one knows how many cases of 'vanishing twins' occur following fertilisation inside the body. There certainly are some, but just how this compares with in vitro fertilisation is unknown.

Another phenomenon that research with IVF has revealed is 'biochemical pregnancies'. These are short-lived pregnancies, that show up as brief hormonal changes, but fail shortly after or during implantation. Treatments for infertility based on hormone stimulation (including IVF) result in slightly more of these early biochemical pregnancies that do not implant as would be expected in a normal cycle. Of those women who had these early tests after embryo transfer at one clinic (Bourn Hall, near Cambridge) between 10 and 15 per cent had 'biochemical pregnancies'[4]. Biochemical pregnancies do occur after 'normal' fertilisation (approximately 6.8 per cent) – but most women would be quite unaware of them.

So, while IVF and ET do allow some infertile women to become pregnant, one less desirable effect is that they can also reveal to others the extent of embryonic loss. Not that this risk is exclusive to those women offered IVF: the introduction of over-the-counter pregnancy testing kits that detect the hormones secreted by the embryo at these earlier stages means that more women are becoming aware of early pregnancy; hence, more women are becoming aware of the extent to which embryos are lost.

Yet it is women seeking treatment for infertility for whom this loss will seem most poignant. Because of the infertility, and because IVF/ET do involve considerable medical control and intervention, doctors are likely to encourage women to have biochemical tests for pregnancy very early, possibly followed by early ultrasound scans to determine whether any embryos have begun to implant. By this time, a woman may well begin to identify herself as having achieved the longed-for pregnancy; this discovery will be made rather earlier than had she achieved fertilisation naturally. Yet many embryos will die at this stage however they were fertilised: knowing one was pregnant, however briefly, may serve only to remind women of the possible pregnancies they have lost.

Embryos in Research

Some embryos created by IVF are destined never to implant and proceed to a pregnancy anyway. Unlike natural embryonic loss, the fate of 'surplus' embryos created through IVF arouses considerable consternation. Because such embryos were created by human intervention, in order to achieve a pregnancy, some people believe that they should not be used for any other purpose; if they are surplus then they could perhaps be frozen for possible transfer to a woman in the future, or they should be allowed to die. What should not happen, according to this view, is that they are used in scientific research.

The arguments put forward in favour of using human embryos for research are not surprising – that research can help to solve problems of infertility (and reveal why so many embryos fail to implant after transfer following IVF, for example); that it may help scientists to develop new contraceptives (such as vaccines); or that it might enable scientists to develop methods of screening embryos for genetic diseases in the laboratory.[5]

The Warnock Committee recommended that embryos could be used in research, subject to a number of reservations – a time limit, for example, and the requirement of 'the informed consent of the couple for whom the embryo was generated'.[6] There were dissident voices on the committee, however. Some members felt that human embryos were special and should not be experimented upon. Banning research will not halt progress in treating infertility, they argued: rather, 'progress can still be made by animal and other experimentation and by the constant endeavour to improve the treatment procedure'.[7] Not surprisingly, the Society for the Protection of Unborn Children (SPUC) was firmly against embryo research in their submissions to Warnock. Equating embryos with children, it argued that 'All experimentation on human zygotes [the fertilised egg], embryos and fetuses should be banned unless for the specific benefit of the particular babies themselves'.[8]

The focus of all this deliberation was the embryo itself and its (potential) moral status. Nowhere (except as part of the couple from whom consent should be obtained) were women specifically part of the debate. Indeed, implicit in SPUC's statement is a disregard for women. Research should 'benefit' that particular 'baby' who, in order to benefit, would have to be transferred into a uterus after being subject to experiment. Feminist concern with embryo research has been quite different; for feminist critics, what is worrying is how those embryos might be obtained.

Many women, as we saw in Chapter Four, may feel quite happy about donating eggs for fertilisation in vitro and subsequent embryo research. Yet as one critic noted, '. . . discussion of research, like that on infertility treatment, does not concede that women's bodies are needed for such research'. Whether embryos are 'surplus' or are created specifically for the purpose, the fact remains that they can be obtained only by extracting eggs (or possibly early embryos) from women. What worries feminist critics is the risk that women may be coerced into donating embryos for research, perhaps during the course of other medical procedures: eggs have been extracted from women undergoing surgery for sterilisation, for example.

On the other hand, should feminists be concerned about the use of embryos in research when those embryos were produced (say) for IVF? Apart from the general objections to IVF procedures that we have already noted, should we worry about the embryo itself? Embryos, in some feminist writing have been viewed as something we possess, as simply a part of the body. So, for example, one article suggests that 'the existence of IVF embryos means researchers have direct access to women's embryos for genetic research'.[9] Robert Edwards, one of the pioneers of IVF, has made a similar point, suggesting that asking for parents' consent implies that the embryo belongs to them and has no rights of its own.[10]

Possession is a tricky argument for feminists to make, however. We have never objected to the use of other human tissues in research; so, if the embryo is just a part of women's bodies, then there is no reason for it to be treated differently. Once it is outside of the body, the embryo assumes a different status; 'there may be legal limitations', argued one critic, about embryos in vitro, 'but the donor has abandoned them and no longer has any rights in them'.[11]

We should certainly be suspicious of claims such as this; it is not the parents who have abandoned the embryo in this formulation (even though it may be 'parents' whose consent is sought), but the mother – 'the donor'. Yet it is not immediately clear why we should claim *possession* of embryos *when they are not inside our bodies*. Women do need to be wary of any attempts to focus exclusively on fetuses, while women's interests and experiences are so obviously ignored. But to claim possession would be to play along with beliefs in the sanctity of the family, to say that someone has rights over an in vitro embryo, simply because it is genetically 'theirs'.

Feminists may dislike the goals of some of the research done, or proposed, on embryos. We may distrust the motives of some of the researchers, or the involvement of commercial concerns. And we may question the ways in which eggs/ embryos are obtained and the effect on women. Yet research on human embryos *as such* should not worry us; they are not, as we have argued, human.

Whose Embryo Is It Anyway? Embryo Donation

If embryos made by IVF can readily be transferred to a woman's womb, they can also be transferred to another woman – another controversial possibility. Perhaps the most celebrated case was that of the woman who gave birth to her own grandchild, after embryo transfer using eggs donated by her daughter. Not surprisingly, traditionalists are opposed to the practice of ET into a woman other than the egg donor, for the simple reason that any resulting children would not 'really' be the children of the woman who bore them.

Donating eggs or embryos – although undoubtedly risky for the women involved – is in one sense no different from donating sperm: both provoke controversy because of the questions they raise for traditional patterns of family relationships, including inheritance, and for the rights of donors. These questions loom larger once the practice of freezing becomes commonplace: by the mid-1980s, women were becoming pregnant with embryos that had been deep-frozen following earlier attempts to harvest their eggs. This has not been particularly controversial in itself so long as the eggs were the woman's own.

The legal systems of most countries recognise certainty in motherhood, even if fatherhood has always been uncertain. Embryo transfer from one woman to another can challenge that certainty.[12] Who, in this case, really *is* the mother? Surrogacy raises related issues, whether or not it also involves transfer of any embryos. The most common form of surrogacy is for a woman to bear a child who has been fathered by the other woman's husband or lover; the surrogate may either have sex with the man, or have artificial insemination. That is, the 'surrogate' provides both the egg and the womb in which the fetus grows. But where the surrogate becomes pregnant through embryo transfer using donated eggs, she provides only the womb; some writers have dubbed this 'womb-leasing', while others more sympathetic to the practice have advocated that it be called 'prenatal adoption'.[13]

The controversy over who is the mother centres on whether we tend to see genetic effects (or the genes themselves) as primary. Indeed, legal battles have been won – and lost – on the grounds that any baby born to a surrogate is not really hers because it is not genetically related to her. It is not surprising, then, that SPUC recommended to the Warnock Committee that 'surrogate motherhood and donor ova should be banned and IVF should be permitted (if at all) only to married couples, with the embryo being transplanted *only to the natural mother*'.[14] Interestingly, the Warnock Committee did not take up this recommendation, but instead advocated that the woman who actually *bore* the child be considered the 'natural' mother – a recommendation now incorporated into draft government legislation in Britain.

Feminist critics have emphasised ways in which various forms of surrogacy might act against the interests of women.[15] There is no doubt that surrogacy of all kinds poses problems; poor women can increasingly be exploited, women who give birth to babies with disabilities may be blamed, and not paid. Increasing emphasis on the notion of fetal personhood may even pose risks of surrogacy being forced on women; Janet Gallagher[16] notes how a proposed statute in Louisiana could enshrine the 'rights of the embryo' even before it is transferred into a woman's body, and speculates how such legislation could result in women being compelled to donate any embryos that are created in vitro but which are surplus to their needs. The 'humanness' of these pre-embryos can be sanctified to the point where they are given the legal right to be implanted in a woman's womb.

It is for these reasons that many feminists (and others) express fear about embryo donation and other forms of surrogacy. On the whole, feminists have not been much concerned with issues of genetic relatedness; most women recognise only too well how often and how easily we step outside that barrier – raising other people's kids, for instance. Indeed, it is for that reason that some feminists have preferred to talk of prenatal adoption to describe surrogacy by embryo donation: ET is, after all, a means of adopting an embryo rather than a baby. And not all forms involve the same degree of medical intervention – one important avenue by which women can be controlled. Juliette Zipper and Selma Sevenhuijsen[17] suggest, for instance, that informal surrogacy arrangements *can* be a form of self-help for women who cannot have a child of their own. Even though embryo donation does require medical intervention, it does not preclude women taking control and using it as a means of helping each other. As such, it could be, potentially, an empowering, rather than oppressive, practice.

Early Pregnancy

Yet the increasing medicalisation of pregnancy can also be oppressive. Some feminist writers fear that it paves the way for greater male control over pregnancy, perhaps even a complete takeover. But, as we have argued, reproductive technologies cannot *yet* give much control over reproduction beyond the stage of implantation: for the moment at least, it is only fertilisation that occurs in the laboratory. Scientists are a long way from being able to make women's bodies completely redundant to reproduction.

The stage over which scientists possibly have the *least* control is the formation of the fetal organs – the development of its brain and nervous system, kidneys, liver, heart and so on. Yet this is a stage when much can go wrong; exposure to drugs, for example, can damage the developing fetal organs permanently (the tragedy of thalidomide is the most familiar example).

By the time the early embryo begins to implant it consists of sheets of cells which have to fold and move as they divide to form different structures. The nervous system begins as a sheet of cells, and folds inwards from the back of the fetus, to form a tube. Occasionally, this inward folding is incomplete, leaving a few cells on the outside: this is the basis of most neural tube defects (NTDs), including spina bifida. Some of these sheets of cells fold outwards from those cells that are destined to become the fetus proper; these move towards, and into, the mother's womb, to create the membranes that will surround the fetus and eventually supply it with nutrients.

Biologically 'the fetus' is continuous with its membranes (which in later pregnancy fill out the entire space of the womb), and with its placenta (to which it is attached by the umbilical cord – another part of the membranes). For that reason, it is usually referred to as the feto-placental unit, to emphasise the continuity between the parts. So when we see photographs of fetuses floating freely in a watery space, the camera is showing us, in effect, the fetus inside part of what it grew itself. We noted earlier how Ros Petchesky has described these photographs as creating images of fetuses devoid of their environment (i.e. the mother): they are also images of fetuses devoid of a part of themselves. What the photography does is to separate that part which *looks* most human, most like a newly born baby, from the rest: yet in reality, it makes no sense biologically to think of it as separate from its membranes. But it does make sense *ideologically*, to create the notion that the fetus is 'really' a miniature person, with full human rights, merely being nourished by the mother's body.

But the womb provides very much more than a warm house and the odd bit of nourishment; the fetus is effectively part of that womb, and in an intimate, two-way relationship with the body of the mother. It is just because of this intimate relationship between the ways that the fetus grows and changes, becoming part of its own surroundings, that it is not easy to control the biological processes of early pregnancy. Basically, this stage of development depends primarily on the capability of the fetus to organise its *own* development. It controls and modifies its own environment, from the beginning of pregnancy when it 'eats' its way into the woman's womb, to the end of pregnancy, when hormonal instructions from the fetus 'tell' the mother's body to begin labour. Throughout the rest of pregnancy, it is in constant biochemical dialogue with the mother's body. Although scientists know some of the details of that dialogue, they are far from understanding it well enough to reproduce it (for further discussion of the idea of ectogenesis, producing babies in the laboratory, see chapter 8).

Producing babies outside the womb is thus a long way off. Still, some medical interventions are possible, which aim to affect the pregnancy. One is to attempt to control events, however, by influencing the mother's behaviour. Women, of course, have had a long history of being made to feel guilty if they do not do certain things during pregnancy – eat the right foods, or take the right amount of rest, for instance. What doctors tell women has possibly changed somewhat over history, but the anxiety and guilt that can be provoked have not.

Various health education campaigns have been directed at pregnant women, aiming, for example, to stop them from smoking during pregnancy. Indeed, so much interest is now taken in encouraging women to have healthy pregnancies, that the notion of 'prepregnancy care' has been invoked: in other words, it is not enough that women look after themselves *during* pregnancy – they must also be personally responsible for maintaining their health prior to conception.[18]

There are, of course, perfectly valid reasons why those concerned with health education, and pregnant women themselves, should want to encourage women to give up smoking during pregnancy, for example: babies born to women who have smoked during pregnancy are smaller, and so more at risk during and after birth. But health education has its own ideology, and it is one which focuses on *individual* solutions. Individuals who do not follow advice have only themselves to blame if they become ill as a result. It is the mother herself who has to make sacrifices like giving up smoking, for the sake of someone else (her baby). As Sue Rodmell has pointed out,[19] the campaign to encourage pregnant women to stop smoking leads to victim-blaming, and ignores the social context of many pregnant women's lives. Most people smoke because they believe it reduces stress – and pregnancy is likely to be stressful if you are struggling to make ends meet.

Moral victim-blaming, though, is only one way in which doctors can exert control over women by stressing their 'responsibility' to look after the health of their 'unborn babies'. A more disturbing trend, particularly evident in the US, is for the courts to intervene to enforce that responsibility. Several courts have ruled, for example, that women *must* undergo caesarian sections, even against their will, to safeguard the life of the unborn child. What, Janet Gallagher has asked, is likely to follow in the wake of such intervention? 'If pregnant women can be legally forced to undergo major surgery,' she asks, 'then why not legal restrictions on prenatal diet, work, sex, sports? After all, such restrictions are certainly less "invasive" or "burdensome" than major surgery. Indeed, why not just lock pregnant women up?'[20] Gallagher's question was followed two years later in 1987 by attempts to take women to court in the US for negligence because they had been taking (illegal) drugs during pregnancy.[21]

Medical control over pregnant women can also be enforced through over-emphasis on the fetus as patient. The fetus is a patient in the sense that its progress is monitored, through prenatal testing (see Chapter Seven) and ultrasound scanning. But it is now becoming a patient in a much more direct sense, through the development of fetal surgery. Doctors have now developed a number of techniques that permit a surgeon to carry out corrective surgery on a fetus before it is born, such as surgical corrections to the urethra. Usually, these are corrections that are necessary for the welfare of the fetus at that stage of its development; in other words, it would die in the womb if the surgical correction was not made. Fetal surgery is unnecessary for conditions that cause no problem before birth, and can be corrected relatively easily afterwards: there is much more risk attached to prenatal surgery. So, if the fetus has a blocked urethra, it cannot get rid of urine and would die if not treated. By contrast, some defects in the heart can be operated on only after the baby is born, because the fetal heart pumps blood somewhat differently to the way it is pumped after the baby is born.

Fetal surgery is not yet common. If it was, many women would no doubt welcome it, as an alternative to either aborting a severely disabled fetus or carrying it to term. But its ready availability could cause problems for women, if fetal rights are given precedence over the rights of mothers. In the US, the courts tend to uphold the principle of fetal rights rather than overtly recognising, as Barbara Katz Rothman suggests, that the best advocate of fetal interests is its mother;[22] rather, maternal and fetal rights are seen as conflicting, and it becomes possible to defend fetal rights *against* the interests of the mother.[23] The mother could then be threatened with legal action if she refused fetal surgery and the fetus then died. Or she could be prosecuted, for instance, for murder or for child abuse.

The threat of legal action is less in Britain, where litigation has, generally, been a last resort. Moreover, when court cases have arisen in Britain (for example, in attempts to make fetuses wards of court and remove them from the mother at birth), they have tended to uphold the very different principle that the best guardian of fetal rights is the mother.

So fetal surgery may be one way in which medical control over women and their pregnancies could increase. Women have already experienced one aspect of the increasing medicalisation of late pregnancy, the 'management' of labour. The induction of labour, like other aspects of giving birth, has become increasingly controlled by doctors. Approximately 9 per cent of all labours were estimated to have involved induction in 1963; by 1984, this had risen to 36 per cent (although there was also a decline in the mid-1970s as the dangers of induction were publicised).

Women's Responses to Technological Control of Pregnancy

One lesson we can learn from this increasing reliance on 'medical management' of labour is the extent to which doctors do turn to new technologies as they arise. Obstetricians have indeed been quick to use new technologies and interventions, from fetal monitors to routine episiotomies, so it might be expected that they would be quick to pick up the newest technologies like IVF. Those feminists who see in obstetric intervention a sinister attempt by a largely male medical profession to control women's bodies may have grounds for their fears; technological childbirth may indeed be a manifestation of that control.

To some feminist critics, the new technologies may allow

that control to be enhanced. As new developments occur, they open up new opportunities for men to intensify their control over women and our reproduction, the argument goes, and we move further down the slippery slope to losing our role in reproduction completely. It can be argued there are ways in which, say, the development of the contraceptive pill, or the development of the techniques of induction have indeed not benefited women, and have contributed to men's control over them; the Pill allows men to coerce women into sex, and inductions have been carried out more for the benefit of hospital staff than for the woman in labour.

Yet, as we pointed out in Chapter Two, that does not mean that these developments are without benefit to women: many women have been freed of the fear of pregnancy by the contraceptive pill, and inductions have often saved the lives of women in labour. And, most important of all, these developments do not mean that women have to accept them passively.

Indeed, the technology of transferring embryos could, in principle, become a part of women's resistance; it could, for example, fit into a world in which women supported and helped each other. Women can, and do, sometimes donate eggs for embryo transfer to close friends or to sisters who are themselves unable to have children because they do not produce viable eggs. Admittedly, this has to be mediated through the medical profession, and women do not have overall control. Still, it does mean that we do not necessarily have to see embryo transfer as inevitably and wholly something which *cannot* benefit women.

What women's struggles around childbirth itself should have taught us is that women can and do resist. From those women who 'vote with their feet' by refusing to turn up for antenatal classes to those women who more actively organise pressure groups to reform the conditions of labour, there has been, as Ann Oakley put it, a consumer revolt. This, she says,

> ... has fought, and continues to fight, against prevailing medical definitions of pregnancy and antenatal care for the very sound reason that what pregnant women have complained about is the capturing of the womb by medical professionals. The consumers' focus has been the reduction of the social and personal experience of pregnancy, and the individuality of pregnant women, to the mechanical image of the womb housed in the body of either a reluctant or compliant patient, and processed on the principle that a no-risk birth is only to be achieved by exposing all wombs and their owners to an identical all-risk monitoring process.[24]

Different women may resist the technological takeover of pregnancy and birth in different ways, depending upon their needs, priorities and social background. Some resist it wholly – the women involved, for example, in the Feminist International Network of Resistance to Reproductive and Genetic Engineering (FINRRAGE). For others, the issue of resistance may be more complex; for some women, the advent of IVF and embryo transfer may open up new possibilities for pregnancy that they experience as empowering, even while they recognise that reproduction has become more medicalised. Many more, especially in poorer countries, will have little or no access to these technologies. But, in thinking about the new technologies, we should remember that women have often resisted medical control. And, presumably, women will resist it in the future.

7. Detecting Genetic Diseases: Prenatal Screening and its Problems

Prenatal diagnosis is the field of medicine that specialises in attempting to detect various 'abnormalities' in the fetus. Only rarely do doctors have an effective treatment to hand – blood transfusions for fetuses whose Rhesus blood type is incompatable with the mother's, for example. But more often there is no treatment, and if the abnormality is deemed severe, many doctors will advise the woman to have an abortion. In this chapter we first discuss the recent history of developments in the field, from the medical profession's point of view, and then go on to consider the impact on women who, despite being on the receiving end of it all, often have little say in the matter.

The past decade has brought major advances in prenatal diagnosis. Doctors have long sought to detect various abnormalities in the fetus, but the daunting complexity of the task has long made the field an esoteric specialism pursued by only a few specialists. Now, advances in the ability both to visualise the fetus, especially through ultrasound, and to analyse its genetic material have made it possible for doctors to talk about 'routine screening', of some or all pregnant women, for many fetal abnormalities.

The medical pioneers of prenatal diagnosis divided defects into crude categories, which are still in use today. The most common serious birth defects are chromosomal abnormalities, such as Down's syndrome. Chromosomes are the structures in the nucleus of a cell that carry the genes (see

Box 7.1. *What Are Genes and Chromosomes?*

Everyone has a unique set of some 100,000 genes, with each cell having its own copy of the set. These genes are coded instructions to tell a cell how to make particular proteins. Roughly speaking, one gene carries the instructions for one protein (or part of one). These proteins, in turn, enable cells to build the body and carry out all the biochemical reactions of life.

The genes themselves are made up of a chemical known as DNA, which in turn is built of a sequence of chemical 'bases' (of which there are four different kinds). These bases act like the letters of the alphabet. The order, or sequence, of these bases spells out a particular protein, rather like the way letters in a particular sequence signify a word.

We inherit our particular mix of genes from our parents – half from each – passed on in the egg and sperm. Thousands of genes are packaged together in large structures known as chromosomes. People normally have 23 pairs of such chromosomes, and inherit one of each pair from each parent. A trained eye can tell the chromosomes apart when they are under the microscope, so they are numbered from 1 to 22 plus the pair of sex chromosomes (XX for females; XY for males).

The uniqueness of our genetic make-up (apart from identical twins) arises largely from the various ways chromosomes are shuffled about as the egg and sperm develop. Through an ingenious process called crossing-over, chromosomes of a pair go through a brief stage where they physically swap bits of themselves to create new combinations of genes on a particular chromosome. Then these newly reconstituted chromosomes of a pair separate, and are sorted at random into a new set of 23 unpaired chromosomes in egg or sperm. When the sex cells meet, the matching chromosomes from each pair up to give 23 pairs again.

box 7.1). People normally have twenty-three pairs of chromosomes, and inherit one of each pair from each parent. Sometimes things go wrong, producing a fetus with three copies of a particular chromosome (as in Down's), or, rarely, only one copy. No one yet understands why an imbalance in the normal complement of chromosomes can produce features such as the characteristic facial structure and mental retardation associated with Down's syndrome children.

Other inborn disorders are known as genetic diseases – or, more precisely, 'single-gene defects' – because a single faulty gene underlies the disease (see box 7.2). Researchers have so far identified about 300 of these disorders, but there may be as many as 1,600. In these cases, a defective gene makes a faulty protein, or sometimes no protein at all. If the normal protein plays a central role in the body, its malfunction causes severe disease. Into this category fall a few relatively common inherited disorders, such as haemophilia, thalassaemia, sickle cell disease, cystic fibrosis and Duchenne muscular dystrophy (see box 7.3). A few single-gene disorders, notably phenylketonuria, or PKU, can be effectively dealt with after birth, through diet for example. People with PKU lack a particular enzyme; undiagnosed, they build up toxins that lead to brain damage. The build-up is prevented if they eat a diet free of a particular amino acid, phenylalanine. Screening for PKU is routine in Britain even though it affects only 1 in 10,000 of the population: newborn babies are tested for PKU by a simple biochemical test on a drop of blood from a pricked heel.

Other disorders in physical development, such as spina bifida and other 'neural tube' defects, tend to be called, rather vaguely, 'congenital' because no one knows what causes them. Still other conditions fall readily into neither category, because they arise from an inherited defect that makes the fetus more vulnerable to something else, such as a harmful chemical in the environment.

Taken together, such serious birth defects occur at a rate of 23 per 1000 births, on a global average. Very few of these

Box 7.2. *What Can Go Wrong?*

Some inborn defects – chromosomal abnormalities – arise when something goes awry with the sorting and swapping of chromosomes. An egg or sperm may end up lacking a particular chromosome, or missing a chunk of one. Most such chromosomal aberrations are lethal at an early age, and cause the embryo to abort spontaneously. In others, such as Down's syndrome, when the embryo has three copies of chromosome 21, instead of two, the fetus often goes to term.

A 'genetic defect' arises if there is a mutation in a single gene. A mutation is a 'mistake' in one or more of the bases that form the building blocks of DNA. The substitution of one base for another, or a deletion or addition of a base, can cause the cell to put together a faulty protein from the garbled instructions, or to make none of that protein at all. A genetic defect can be fatal, or harmless, depending upon what that protein normally does, or whether there is another, normal gene that can compensate for the mutated one.

Genes come in pairs, one at equivalent spots on a pair of chromosomes. These genes may be identical or slightly different variants. If one normal gene can do enough work for two, we say that the gene (or the disease) is 'recessive' – its presence is hidden by the normal gene inherited on the other chromosome. People with just one copy of such a recessive gene are said to be 'carriers'; the disease itself will appear in their children only if their reproductive partners are carriers too. A 'dominant' gene is the reverse – even a single copy of a defective version is enough to bring on the disease. Most genetic diseases, such as cystic fibrosis, are recessive. Huntington's chorea is an example of a dominant one.

There is a further complication, caused by genes on the sex chromosomes. The Y chromosome carries a gene that determines maleness – called the 'testes determining factor' – but little else. In the absence of the Y chromosome (or more specifically, without the testes determining factor), the fetus will develop as a female. Women carry two copies of the X chromosome (while men have only one), and the X chromo-

> some is packed with genes. A consequence of this arrangement is that, in a boy, a recessive gene on an X chromosome acts like a dominant (since it is alone) and invariably shows itself in a man, but not in a woman. The woman will 'carry' the hidden recessive gene, however, and invariably pass it on to her sons. Muscular dystrophy and haemophilia are two examples of diseases passed on in this way, through the X chromosome.

disorders can be treated effectively, and they account for about a third of admissions to paediatric wards in the West, and a large proportion of childhood deaths. Some epidemiologists argue that infant mortality cannot fall below the 20 per 1000 mark, now achieved by Japan and most Western countries, unless we can treat, or prevent, severe chronic disease with a genetic basis.

Until recently, doctors interested in the plethora of ill-understood disorders of the developing fetus have had only rather primitive ways of studying them. The work of cell biologists in the 1950s and 1960s led to the first breakthrough – the ability to study a fetus's chromosomes. These scientists – 'cytogeneticists' – perfected ways of detecting extra chromosomes in fetal cells. Staining dividing cells with special dyes creates distinctive bands on the chromosomes that enable an experienced eye to tell the various chromosomes apart, and to detect small missing portions (deletions). Cytogeneticists photograph dividing cells, cut out the individual chromosomes and arrange them in an orderly group portrait, known in the trade as a 'karyotype'.

Medical cytogenetics came of age in 1959. A French geneticist, Jerome Lejeune, discovered that children with Down's syndrome have three, rather than the normal two, copies of chromosome 21. Lejeune's discovery caused a great stir, as researchers of the time, and a eugenically minded population at large, had long suspected that 'feeblemindedness' was inherited, passed on from 'inferior' parents to their offspring.[1] Even liberal-minded scientists were excited by the notion that we might begin to discover the genetic basis of many human ills. The search began for other abnormalities of the chromosomes, and for a way of diagnosing chromosomal aberrations before birth. Doctors soon refined a technique for harvesting fetal cells – dubbed 'amniocentesis'. It became possible to diagnose disorders such as Down's syndrome in the second trimester of pregnancy.

In amniocentesis, doctors extract some of the amniotic fluid that surrounds the fetus, via a needle through the woman's abdomen. This technique exploits the fact that the fetus sheds some of its own cells into the fluid, making the procedure a sort of fetal urine sample. The idea of diagnosing fetal defects in this way is not new; it was first suggested some fifty years ago. But it is only in the past twenty years that the technique has become a standard procedure in the obstetrics wards of the developed world. In England and Wales, for instance, between 2 and 3 per cent of pregnant women now have amniocentesis.

In Britain, doctors' enthusiasm for prenatal diagnosis was fuelled by the passing of the Abortion Act of 1967, which legalised the termination of affected fetuses, for the medics felt that there was no point in diagnosing something that they could do nothing about. Over the next two decades, women's magazines and obstetricians joined forces to spread the word, focusing particularly on amniocentesis for Down's syndrome which occurs in the West at the rate of about 1 in 750 live births, and is the most common cause of mental retardation.

The campaign was a success, by some counts. Skirting the question of whether screening for Down's syndrome is a good idea, doctors forged ahead with the task of informing the public about the availability of amniocentesis. Many lay people now know that older women, especially those over forty, run a higher risk of having a baby with Down's, and doctors are most likely to offer the test to older pregnant women.

Nonetheless, despite the success of the 'educational' campaign, amniocentesis for Down's syndrome remains a bit of an embarrassment for the advocates of prenatal diagnosis. Even within Britain, amniocentesis is not universally available on the NHS, and some regions have different age cut-offs than others – thirty-eight versus thirty-five, for instance. The availability of amniocentesis has also had little impact on the number of Down's syndrome children born. This is not because most women over thirty-five or forty are rejecting the test or generally refusing to abort affected fetuses, nor even because doctors fail to offer them the test. Rather, amniocentesis for older women most at risk has little impact because 80 per cent of Down's syndrome babies are born to younger women, under thirty-five. Even though younger women are individually at lower risk, they have so many more of each year's crop of babies that they also have more Down's syndrome babies, in direct proportion.

Why not offer amniocentesis to all women then? For a start, the test can lead to the spontaneous abortion of a fetus. Much debate among medics centres on the precise risk of miscarriage – some studies suggest it is as low as 0.5 per cent (1 in 200), others as high as 1.7 per cent. The expertise of the practitioner, and the technique used, such as the size of the needle and the availability of ultrasound, probably account for some of the disagreement.

Health economists also argue that it is not cost effective to screen all women; because the individual risk for younger women is so low, large numbers would have to be tested for each Down's syndrome fetus detected, so the cost becomes astronomical. Doctors also argue that testing younger women as a matter of course would be unethical, because the risk of producing a spontaneous abortion from the test may be higher than the risk of Down's syndrome in younger women. This seems a sensible argument on the face of it, but makes a dubious assumption: that all women will give the two probabilities the same weight, so as to equate the risk of spontaneous abortion with the risk of having a Down's baby. Depending upon their beliefs, experiences and circumstances, individual women may well balance the risks very differently.

Another drawback to amniocentesis is its timing. The amniotic fluid contains too few fetal cells before about sixteen weeks of pregnancy. Even then, amniocentesis retrieves only a few fetal cells, so technicians have to grow them in the laboratory for two weeks or more to have enough dividing ones to karyotype. It can take a month or more to get the results, forcing those women whose test results suggest something is 'wrong' to contemplate a late abortion, with all its emotional traumas and physical risks.

Amniocentesis can pick up defects other than Down's, however, notably other chromosomal aberrations (see box 7.3) and a few rare 'inborn errors of metabolism'. For instance, David Brock and his colleagues in Edinburgh have developed a biochemical assay of enzymes in the amniotic fluid that is a test for cystic fibrosis. It detects 90 per cent of affected fetuses at high risk of inheriting the defective gene, but, as is often the case with such tests, is not sensitive enough for use as a general screen. Amniocentesis has also long been used to detect the failure of the spinal column to close – the so-called neural tube defects, such as spina bifida. Neural tube defects occur in about 1 in every 1000 live births, among Celts and Sikhs in particular, and so are relatively common. The causes of these birth defects are varied, and largely unknown, and for some reason are more common in Europe than in Asia or Africa; and in Britain they are more common in Northern Ireland than in London. Numbers have been falling in Britain since 1972, perhaps because of better nutrition. (There is some evidence that vitamins taken by the mother before and around conception may help to prevent these defects.) But the incidence of neural tube defects is also falling in impoverished areas of northern Britain, where

Box 7.3. *Chromosomal Abnormalities*

Down's syndrome is the most common aberration of the chromosomes, but an analysis of fetal cells can reveal other anomalies. The question is then, what should be done with this information? No one is certain about the effects of some of these other abnormalities.

Chromosomes other than the chromosome 21 involved in Down's syndrome may have an extra copy. Most of these abnormalities grossly distort development in some way and children often die as infants or during the first few years of life. Cytogeneticists can also detect breaks in chromosomes, or missing bits. In such cases, doctors often find it impossible to predict whether the child will be, say, severely mentally retarded or only mildly so. Finally, there may be an abnormality of the sex chromosomes, producing a range of symptoms in the child.

For example, a child with a single X chromosome (XO), known as Turner's syndrome, has female genitalia but is usually sterile. A person with XXY has male genitalia, but small testes, and is sterile – a syndrome known as Klinefelter's. It occurs once in every 400 to 600 male births, while Turner's is much rarer, occurring once in about every 3,500 female births. Since the 1950s many other combinations have been discovered. For instance, one in about every 1,000 newborn males has XYY sex chromosomes. They seem to be taller than the average man, may have severe acne, but otherwise seem 'normal'. Controversy rages over whether men with XYY tend to be more aggressive, after several studies found that men of this sex chromosome constitution are somewhat more likely to be incarcerated in mental-penal institutions than men with XY sex chromosomes. In the mid-1970s, a group of American cytogeneticists and psychiatrists tried to begin a mass screening programme to detect XYY males in the general population, although they eventually abandoned the scheme under pressure from civil rights activists.

The sex chromosome anomalies in particular present a
(Continued overleaf)

> dilemma to the medical authorities. Should they tell the parents, and let them decide whether to terminate the pregnancy? Or would the mere knowledge that something was 'wrong', such as an XYY condition, lead parents to treat their child differently?
>
> Some cytogeneticists feel that the way to deal with the problem of chromosomal abnormalities is to collect more information on how affected fetuses turn out, so that they can give parents better advice. A central registry in Edinburgh, for instance, collates case histories, and is following the development of XYY boys to see if they are more aggressive than most. Genetic counsellors tend to argue that women should be informed of the risk of finding such sex chromosome abnormalities beforehand, and asked whether they wish to be told about them. In desperation, some clinicians have even suggested that we should devise a way of karyotyping a cell (analysing its chromosomes) without looking at its sex chromosomes – and so circumvent the problem altogether.

the dramatic decline has gone hand in hand with growing unemployment and fall in living standards.[2]

Against this background of mysterious cause, the prenatal diagnosis of neural tube defects has bloomed. Developed some fifteen years ago, its appeal is the simplicity of the first screening test: an analysis of the mother's blood. A tell-tale sign of an open spinal column in the developing fetus is an abnormal amount of alpha fetoprotein, produced by the fetal liver. The fetus normally excretes this substance into the amniotic fluid and a tiny amount enters the mother's bloodstream. High levels of alpha fetoprotein (AFP), however, suggest that something is wrong. Doctors may then offer to perform an amniocentesis to check the levels of AFP in the amniotic fluid. In the past few years, however, obstetricians have tended to use high-resolution ultrasonography, instead of amniocentesis, to confirm the presence of a neural tube defect.[3]

In England and Wales, some 60 per cent of pregnant

women now have a blood test for AFP as a standard part of their antenatal care, but numbers vary dramatically from region to region (from almost all women in Oxford and North East Thames to almost none in East Anglia). In theory, they are told about the purpose of the test and asked for their consent. In practice, the test is often performed routinely, without informed consent.

There are technical problems with the 'maternal serum' AFP test, too. It is not foolproof, because there are marked changes in the levels of AFP during pregnancy, and between individual women. A worrying blood test may well turn out to be a false alarm, after an unnecessary amniocentesis. Or the test may falsely reassure women that all is well. Levels of AFP in the mother's blood can detect only about 60 per cent of fetuses with spina bifida, for instance. Furthermore, the severity of neural tube defects varies greatly, and it is not always easy to tell them apart, even with ultrasound scans. In about half of the cases, the tube is open at the top and the babies are born with a very rudimentary brain, or no brain at all (anencephaly). These babies invariably die around birth. Spina bifida occurs if the opening of the neural tube is along the spine, exposing some of the neural column. Babies with this condition are paralysed from the opening down. Sometimes these babies also develop hydrocephaly, when fluid accumulates in the head to cause brain damage.

Despite the disadvantages inherent in AFP-testing, it is growing in popularity in the US. There, doctors are beginning to offer women the test fuelled by fears that, if they do not, they will be sued by patients who have an affected child. American commentators have already expressed concern that 'whether a prenatal screening is offered may depend as much on the patient's health insurance and the physician's perception of possible legal liability as on the physician's view of the patient's welfare'.[4]

Controversy over the role of AFP testing has increased in the past few years, since several groups of researchers published data suggesting that *low* levels of AFP in a woman's blood seem to indicate that the fetus may have Down's syndrome. Using blood tests, followed by amniocentesis, doctors might be able to detect between 20 and 30 per cent of Down's syndrome fetuses, in women of all ages.[5]

Some argue that this is hardly a satisfactory screening test – a negative test would by no means be reassuring. American doctors have pointed out: 'The high prevalence of false positive results is a problem, since the women so identified were subjected to time-consuming, costly, and emotionally traumatic procedures.'[6] Estimates suggest that if screening were adopted throughout the US, 150,000 women under 35 would undergo amniocentesis. Because the ability of AFP to predict Down's is low, widespread amniocentesis would probably mean that more normal fetuses were lost because of the test than fetuses with Down's discovered by screening.

But some researchers, such as Howard Cuckle of St Bartholomew's Hospital in London, argue that a combination of a woman's age and the AFP levels in her blood gives a better estimate of her risk of a Down's syndrome birth.[7] Doctors could then detect some 35 per cent of affected fetuses, by doing an amniocentesis test on just 5 per cent of pregnant women. Some women in their early thirties and late twenties could be identified as being at high risk because they have low levels of AFP in their blood, and referred for amniocentesis, while some older women could be excluded on account of high levels, says Cuckle. In the future, other biochemical screening tests for Down's may improve detection rates. Determining levels of the hormone oestriol, combined with age and levels of maternal AFP, could 'yield a detection rate of 45 per cent for an amniocentesis rate of 5 per cent. Using age alone, 15 per cent of women would require amniocentesis to achieve such high detection,' says Cuckle.

The debate continues, and in the US, the desirability of universal blood tests to measure AFP levels in all pregnant women, to screen for neural tube defects and Down's, remains under question. The American College of Obstetricians and Gynecologists, on the advice of its lawyers, now urges doctors to offer women an AFP test for neural tube defects, but to tell women that using the results to detect Down's as well is still 'investigational' and leave them to try to make sense of it all.[8] But some states have gone further. Since April 1986, California has required obstetricians to offer a blood test for AFP, on a voluntary basis. The state provides a brochure that explains birth defects and the screening programme in simple language. Women are then asked to sign a 'statement of informed consent/refusal', and about half agree to the test. The test itself costs $40 and is covered by most health insurance schemes, as are the costs of amniocentesis. But a woman has to pay for an abortion of an affected fetus if she wants one.

Perhaps the most important point to emerge from decades of prenatal diagnosis is that, broadly speaking, it has not been a roaring success. Amniocentesis late in pregnancy, followed by laborious and expensive karyotyping (analysis of chromosomes), or biochemical tests for neural tube defects, are not the stuff of mass screening. Such procedures cannot support a 'search and destroy' mission against severe congenital deformity and genetic disease throughout the population. Ultrasound too is still too primitive to catch many physical defects (see box 7.4). 'Fetoscopy' performed at seventeen weeks of gestation or more uses a fine fibre-optic tube to examine the fetus visually. But it is hazardous, even in experienced hands, and causes miscarriages about 4 per cent of the time.[9] It is mostly used for extracting a fetal blood sample or a bit of liver or skin to detect rare inborn errors of metabolism in couples already known to be at risk of having an affected child.

Despite the disappointing track record of prenatal diagnosis to date, two recent developments have generated great enthusiasm among clinicians working in the field: the prospect of diagnosis at the level of the gene, combined with a new way of sampling fetal tissue, early in pregnancy. It is now even possible to screen embryos for some genetic

> **Box 7.4.** *Ultrasound*
>
> Attempts to 'visualise' the fetus are fraught with difficulties and are not yet a great success. It began badly and in some ways is still primitive. In the early days of X-rays there was a brief medical vogue for popping pregnant women under the machines to look at the fetus – a fashion abruptly abandoned once radiologists realised the dangers of thereby causing a 'defect' themselves.
>
> Ultrasound is now the technology of choice for such purposes. It is apparently safe, although there are still debates about whether we have enough information to assess its possible effects on young embryos in the long term. In experienced hands, an 'anomaly scan' at about twenty weeks can undoubtedly detect many major congenital defects, such as anencephaly, where no brain develops. Yet interpretation is all, given the fuzzy images of ultrasound, and many medics are sceptical of some of the claims made by ultrasound enthusiasts. For instance, some sonographers advocate replacing blood tests for AFP with ultrasound scans to detect spina bifida. Other researchers claim to be able to detect 82 per cent of Down's fetuses during the second trimester through ultrasound.
>
> Yet other doctors stress how misleading ultrasound can be, finding false positives (i.e. results that appear to indicate a positive result for, say, spina bifida, when the fetus is normal) commonplace. In Britain, the Medical Research Council is conducting a trial to try to assess the strengths and weaknesses of diagnostic ultrasound. So far, it has most proven its worth only in a more humble role, guiding the procedures of amniocentesis and the new technique of chorionic villus sampling (CVS) and retrieval of eggs in IVF. At the moment, antenatal clinics rely on ultrasound scans mostly to check the age of the fetus and to spot twins.

diseases in the laboratory, before a pregnancy has even begun.

What is strikingly new is the ability of doctors, teamed with scientists, to diagnose many of the genetic diseases that arise as a result of a single faulty gene. Advances in the techniques of molecular biology have made this possible.[10] Already, in theory, researchers can detect some forty single gene defects in a fetus.

The molecular diagnosis relies on one of two basic approaches. The test may detect the presence of the faulty gene itself, if we know what it is. Or it may detect some other gene nearby – usually a harmless gene that is interesting only because it is physically near enough on the chromosome to the as-yet-unknown faulty one to act as a 'genetic marker' (rather like identifying a house because you know what the neighbouring one looks like).

The first approach works only if researchers know exactly where the faulty gene is, among the thousands strung along the various chromosomes, and have also determined its precise chemical structure. It is no small task to locate a disease-causing gene, and scores of molecular biologists all over the world are now trying to 'map' them. Once discovered, however, the genes can be readily mass produced in the laboratory. Then, researchers can use the gene as a 'probe' that will bind to its match in the DNA extracted from a sample of someone's cells and so directly reveal whether that person has that particular faulty gene.

The second approach to molecular diagnosis is less direct, but it means that you do not have to know the exact location or chemical make-up of the faulty gene. In this approach, researchers use marker genes that are physically near to the gene of interest, as the genes are arranged on a chromosome. (A close marker gene is said to be 'linked' to the disease-causing gene.)

Take cystic fibrosis (CF) as an example. Researchers know that the gene responsible is on chromosome number 7; in 1988 they did not yet know its exact location, but had found several genes that were physically very close to the defective gene on the chromosome. These acted as 'genetic markers' to trace the inheritance of a defective gene, sitting on a particular chromosome, through several generations.

Parents who are carriers of the disease have one chromosome 7 that bears a copy of the CF gene, and one normal chromosome 7. The trick is to establish which chromosome is which (you can't tell by looking), so that you can determine which the fetus has inherited: the fetus may be affected with CF (with a chromosome 7 bearing the CF gene from each parent), normal (receiving a normal chromosome 7 from each) or a carrier itself (with a CF-bearing chromosome 7 from one parent and a normal one from the other).

To make such a diagnosis, researchers have to do 'family studies'. First, they extract samples of DNA (from blood cells) from as many members of a family as possible, including grandparents and parents if possible. Then, the researchers analyse the DNA to identify the genetic markers near the CF gene. Ideally, each chromosome 7 belonging to the mother and father will carry a different variant of the marker gene, so that the researchers can tell the markers, and thus the chromosomes, apart. If you are lucky and the family is informative, you can pinpoint the disease, or its absence, to the inheritance of a particular set of chromosomes, distinguished by which variant of the genetic marker they carry.

Clearly this approach has several disadvantages. It works only if father, mother and sibs, and preferably grandparents, are alive and give permission for their DNA to be analysed. Even then, the family may not be 'informative'; the test fails if everyone has the same form of the marker gene because you cannot tell which chromosomes bear the defective gene. The probe also has to be very close to the disease gene, to map accurately the inheritance of the faulty gene. The more distant the marker gene is on the chromosome, the greater the chance that the marker will give misleading results because it has become separated from the disease gene. This can happen when chromosomes swap bits as the sex cells are formed (a process known as crossing over: see box 7.1).

Researchers in San Francisco were among the first to use

DNA in prenatal diagnosis, to detect a fetus with sickle cell anaemia, in 1978.[11] They extracted DNA from fetal cells retrieved by amniocentesis. In 1982 researchers in Oxford broke new ground by diagnosing beta-thalassaemia in the first trimester of pregnancy, by a new technique for extracting fetal cells, known as chorionic villus sampling (CVS).[12] Since then, scores of single-gene defects have been diagnosed by the technique. It now often takes just a few months to take the discovery of a new disease-causing gene or a new genetic marker from the laboratory into clinical practice, in the form of prenatal diagnosis.

We know most about the genetic disorders affecting haemoglobin, the complex protein that carries oxygen in the blood. Several genes are involved in making the different parts of the complete protein, and defects in the different genes cause different forms of diseases, such as several forms of thalassaemia and sickle cell anaemia. Many of these diseases can now be diagnosed in a fetus using the first approach – direct gene probes.

Gene probes that focus on the defective gene itself are also available for a disease called alpha-antitrypsin deficiency, which can lead to severe cirrhosis of the liver and emphysema (a lung disease) in childhood, for two types of haemophilia and for phenylketonuria (PKU). Duchenne's muscular dystrophy joined this list in 1987, as researchers at last pinpointed the defective gene at the root of the disorder. The gene responsible for cystic fibrosis was discovered as recently as 1989.

Researchers know less about other genetic diseases, but can detect several via linked probes in some family studies: these include Becker muscular dystrophy, myotonic dystrophy, Huntington's disease, Alzheimer's disease and even, by some accounts, schizophrenia.

Earlier Screening? The Development of CVS

Our growing ability to detect genetic diseases using DNA-based tests has fostered the development of CVS. Invented

Box 7.5. Why Defective Genes?

Superimposed on the vast genetic continuity that make people a single species are slight regional differences. Geneticists find variations in how common a particular gene is – differences in 'gene frequency' – in different parts of the world.

Many of these genes that vary between regions in their frequency produce harmless differences in some physical characteristic. Many arise by chance and are of interest to geneticists studying populations only because they help them to chart the movement of groups of people through history, or measure the degree of inbreeding. Certain blood groups, for instance, are more common in Italy than in Britain.

But regions of the world can also differ in the prevalence of certain genetic diseases. For instance, Tay-Sachs is a severe disorder of the nervous system that develops when a child is just a few years old, and leads to death in childhood. It is more common among Jews of Eastern European origin. Cystic fibrosis is fairly common among whites of northern European origin, but not in other groups, while thalassaemia is widespread in Mediterranean countries, Africa and the Indian subcontinent. Sickle cell disease is more common among people of central African origins.

How can we explain such regional variations? Sometimes a certain genetic disease is more common in a particular group of people by chance; a mutation arose at random and then spread among a group of people who inter-married. Other disorders appear to have been perpetuated because being a carrier (with a single copy of the defective recessive gene) confers some advantage in a particular environment, and so people who carry the gene reproduce successfully and pass the gene on. Carriers of thalassaemia and sickle cell disease, for example, are apparently more resistant to malaria.

Evidence is growing that most of the genes that we now associate with death or severe disease may have been beneficial to the population as a whole in different circumstances. For instance, a genetic propensity to develop diabetes or to put on weight is harmful in the West where sugary food is

> abundant. But the same genes may have been an aid to survival in times of famine, or when people were eating a Neolithic diet. Similarly, a gene that leads to iron poisoning in some middle-aged men in our society may have once prevented women of child-bearing age from developing anaemia.
>
> Hence genes have meaning, in terms of good or bad, only in a particular context, made up of other genes and of the environment. The genetic mix that we each inherit is the result of generations of human evolution. In fact, everyone carries 'bad' genes in one form or another and is at risk of producing a child with a genetic disorder. Furthermore, things can go awry in the development of sperm and egg to create new mutations or chromosomal defects. To make matters even more unpredictable, many congenital malformations – ranging from cleft palate to spina bifida – probably have some genetic basis, complexly intermeshed with environmental factors.

in China, this technique was refined in Britain and the US in the early 1980s at elite medical centres. To date, more than 17,000 women throughout the world at some ninety centres have had CVS.[13] In Europe, CVS was developed on women who were about to have an elective abortion. In the US, many states have banned such research so doctors interested in the techniques tried them first on women who wanted to keep the pregnancy; apparently, some women lost them as a result.[14]

The appeal of the test is the fact that it is a way of obtaining fetal tissue early on in pregnancy, from about nine to eleven weeks. This means that an affected fetus could be aborted much earlier than the twenty-four weeks or so necessitated by amniocentesis.

In chorionic villus sampling, doctors remove a bit of tissue from the portion of the placenta that is contributed by the fetus. Chorionic villi are finger-like projections of the chorion, the outer membrane of the gestation sac surrounding the fetus. Typically, using a flexible cannula or rigid forceps inserted through the woman's cervix, doctors snip off a few villi to obtain enough cells to test. Ultrasound imaging is essential to enable doctors to guide the instruments to the right spot, avoiding blood vessels, the fetus itself, and so on.

The fetal cells harvested by CVS can be examined directly; there are sufficient dividing cells in the villi to test immediately for chromosomal abnormalities such as Down's. This gives CVS a big advantage over amniocentesis, where technicians must grow fetal cells in the laboratory for several weeks before they can analyse any chromosomes. Equally important, these villus cells are also usually plentiful enough to enable biologists to extract DNA to test for genetic diseases such as thalassaemia.[15] If not, a technique developed in 1988 known as the polymerase chain reaction enables researchers to make more copies ('amplify') a portion of DNA, so ensuring that there is enough to analyse.[16]

Many people predict that chorionic villus sampling will soon largely replace amniocentesis. Because it can be performed early in pregnancy, it removes the need for late abortions in many cases. But the safety of the new technique compared to amniocentesis is still uncertain. Clinical trials in Europe, Canada and the US suggest that about 2 per cent of fetuses spontaneously abort after the test, compared to 1 per cent or less after amniocentesis. But the apparently higher risk of spontaneous abortion after CVS probably reflects the fact that the test is carried out much earlier in pregnancy – many of the fetuses might have miscarried anyway.[17] At the time of writing, further clinical trials comparing the two techniques are still under way in Britain and Europe. So far, there has been no obvious rise in congenital abnormalities in babies born after CVS. But specialists point out that it will be many years before we know definitely that there are no additional risks to the fetus from the placental sampling.[18] The early ultrasound scans needed to guide the procedure could also conceivably present a hazard to the young fetus, but so far there is no evidence from either epidemiological or laboratory studies to suggest that the scans do harm.[19] The new technique, especially the transcervical route, may pose greater risks of infection to women; in a few cases, women have developed severe life-threatening infections after CVS. Sampling through the woman's abdominal wall, as in amniocentesis, offers less risk of infection because the skin (through which the needle passes) harbours fewer potentially infective bacteria and viruses than does the cervix. Other doctors argue that the abdominal route takes longer and harvests fewer cells, but its medical supporters claim that it has the added advantage of being 'more dignified' for the woman.

This transabdominal route may also make CVS feasible in the second trimester of pregnancy – further supplanting amniocentesis. Early on in pregnancy, doctors performing CVS extract a part of the chorion destined to degenerate at around twelve weeks of pregnancy, but subsequent forays have shown that it is possible to sample another region of the chorion later in pregnancy. CVS via a transabdominal route is now becoming the norm between twelve weeks, the latest date for cervical CVS, and about fifteen weeks, the earliest for amniocentesis.

A major disadvantage of CVS, however, is that it cannot diagnose neural tube defects such as spina bifida. Existing tests are based on the detection in the amniotic fluid of high levels of AFP leaking from the fetus's open spinal column. Similarly, CVS is less reliable than amniocentesis for detecting some metabolic conditions. Another problem with CVS, still unresolved by specialists working in the field, is the high incidence of cells with different chromosomes, with some cells having, say, an extra X or Y chromosome, while the others are normal.[20] If the fetus really did have a patchwork of genetically different cells, some with normal sets of chromosomes and some with something wrong, researchers would call the fetus a 'mosaic'. What is worrying about the chorionic villus sampling is that sometimes it is *only* the villi that are such a mosaic: the fetus itself is normal. The question is, how is one to tell whether the chromosome anomalies one finds are really a harmless 'pseudomosaic' or represent a genuine mosaic fetus?

The placenta is rather odd, biologists now think; it seems to have an inherent tendency to generate cells with chromosomal abnormalities. The danger is that this ill-understood quirk of nature could lead to the abortion of a normal fetus on mistaken grounds. One way to reduce the risk is to advise a woman to wait and have an amniocentesis later in pregnancy, to double check the fetus's chromosomes. Hence, as some cytogeneticists have pointed out, the risk of a misleading 'pseudomosaic' threatens to limit the utility of widespread genetic screening by CVS. When a woman is at low risk of carrying a fetus with a chromosomal abnormality such as Down's – because she is young, say – the risk of diagnosing a mosaic fetus falsely may be unacceptably high.

Ethics and Politics

Prenatal diagnosis has already stimulated considerable debate, among professionals as well as feminists. For not even all doctors agree. One highly respected African doctor, for example, wrote to the *British Medical Journal* in 1984 to denounce abortion on the grounds of genetic disease: 'I was born, in the Krobo tribe, with extra digits – a Mendelian dominant condition [i.e. due to a dominant gene] with a 1 per cent incidence at birth in Ghana. Had I been born a few miles southeast across the Volta river, there would have been great rejoicing because local tribesmen had it that I was destined to be rich. If my mother had given birth to me a few miles northwest beyond the hills, I would not be here to write to you – I would have been drowned soon after birth. Fortunately, the Krobos were neutral to extra digits but, until the government forbade the practice, some tribal elders took it onto themselves to decide which genes ought to be allowed to survive . . .' Other doctors take the view, as David Weatherall of the John Radcliffe Hospital in Oxford puts it, that 'the potential parents of genetically abnormal children should have the right to decide what kind of children they bring into the world'.[21]

Unfortunately, little time or money has been spent trying to find out what women think of it all. Few studies tell us about the attitudes and experience of women in screening. Most ask in general terms whether patients were happy with the service they received. Such surveys tell us little, as many studies have shown that people in such situations tend to express satisfaction with whatever form of health care they receive.

Research by Wendy Farrant in Britain points to the fundamental inadequacy of provision by the health service for women undergoing prenatal diagnosis.[22] Everything from emotional support to information on the medical techniques used is insufficient, she finds. These findings reduce women's autonomy, and ability to make free and informed choices, even if women actually want the option of prenatal diagnosis.

Sally Macintyre, director of the Medical Research Council's medical sociology unit at the University of Glasgow, has pointed out the need for descriptive studies that explore what actually happens to women in genetic screening programmes.[23] Most women studied have been screened and correctly given an 'all-clear' for whatever condition they are being screened, or have had a handicapped baby and are now asked if they want screening for subsequent pregnancies. But we cannot extrapolate the experiences of these women to others. How can we compare the reassurances of the true negative, of knowing that your baby is really 'all right' with the anguish of a false negative – being told it is, and then finding out it isn't – or a false positive or a miscarriage after the test? How can we decide 'what women want'? Does the question even make sense, given the constraints on women's choices? There is a widespread tendency in the medical profession to stereotype women, says Macintyre. We need to understand, she says, that screening creates many different subgroups with different experiences – not all women are the same, nor are they all in the same situation. For instance, a woman who elects to terminate a wanted pregnancy because of a mistaken diagnosis is not readily comparable to a woman having an amniocentesis for Down's syndrome who later miscarries a normal fetus. A woman's age and the size of the existing family may also make a big difference to her feelings, say, about the risk of miscarriage after testing.

A younger woman may feel more able to abort an affected fetus or risk miscarriage, and start again; an older woman may fear for her continued fertility. Meanwhile, doctors argue over the age at which women should be offered amniocentesis for Down's and other chromosomal abnormalities, and usually see it as a medical question. For most hospitals, the lower age limit is between thirty-five and thirty-seven, but some groups in Britain say that young women are increasingly likely to ask for the test. In one survey of some seventy women in Leeds, reported in *The Lancet*, 70 per cent of the women 'regarded a Down's birth as worse than a miscarriage after amniocentesis', and so would have accepted amniocentesis on average even if the risk was higher.[24] But the answers ranged from those women who would always refuse amniocentesis to those who would have it even if the risk of a Down's baby were as low as 1 in 20,000. The doctors conclude 'that the current almost universal failure to perform amniocentesis on women under thirty-five and the high acceptance rates over thirty-five are probably not based on a correct measure of women's values – a sizeable proportion, not merely a hyperanxious minority, would like the procedure at a lower risk'.

The data on how women feel about chorionic villus sampling are equally sparse. The Medical Research Council in Britain has organised a 'randomised' trial to compare the safety of amniocentesis and chorionic villus sampling. To work as a controlled trial, and so ensure that any differences in the results are not due to some differences between the women who choose CVS or amniocentesis, the researchers randomly assign women agreeing to participate in the study to one or other of the tests. Some commentators complain that this kind of trial is an infringement of individual choice, while the medics argue that we cannot know whether one test is better than the other unless we do proper studies, and that it is unethical not to do so.

The point, in the context of a discussion of 'what women want', is that researchers had already tried to set up trials comparing the two techniques without randomly assigning women, by letting them choose after hearing the pros and cons of each test. The peculiar result was that in London, everyone wanted CVS, while in Oxford, everyone wanted amniocentesis.[25] This may well reflect in part biases in the way women were advised about the two tests, but even so it seems that we cannot predict how 'women' as a whole will feel about the two tests. In a small survey of sixty-five women in Oxford, those most at risk of having a genetically abnormal child, because of their age or because they had already had an affected pregnancy, almost invariably wanted CVS. Those women at lower risk requested CVS or amniocentesis at a ratio of 2 to 1. Barbara Katz Rothman, in her excellent book, *The Tentative Pregnancy*, has argued that the fact that CVS can be done earlier than amniocentesis is not necessarily a boon for all women.[26] The earlier diagnosis spares some women the pain associated with late diagnosis (and hence a possible late abortion), but six times as many will have to share the pain of a positive diagnosis, she claims, if it is done much earlier: and many of these would have miscarried anyway.

The very existence of screening programmes creates anxiety in women and further 'medicalises' pregnancy. For instance, most women will have had no experience of neural tube defects, so being given a test for them arouses new fears. And Barbara Katz Rothman describes how the very existence of prenatal diagnosis puts a woman into a horrifying dilemma. If she has amniocentesis for Down's, say, she must risk damaging a normal fetus, and then decide, if something is 'wrong', whether to abort a wanted child. Throughout the long wait for the results, she must regard her pregnancy as 'tentative' – even after she has felt the fetus move. Even a 'reassuring' result on amniocentesis may fail to allay a woman's fears, Rothman says, because it has raised the fears in the first place, and cannot pretend to diagnose all possible defects.

Even crude psychometric tests designed to measure people's levels of anxiety demonstrate the intensity of women's feeling. For instance, Bryan Hibbard and his colleagues at the University of Wales College of Medicine found that when women were told that they had raised levels of AFP in their blood (a potential sign of a neural tube defect), they scored an average of 59 on an anxiety scale running from 20 to 80.[27] People in medical wards of the hospital scored 42, and people with anxiety disorders a mere 49. A normal result after amniocentesis lowered their anxiety only to 37. Hibbard's study also reveals the flaw in the 'no news is good news' approach, adopted by some clinics who inform women of the results only if there is something wrong. Two weeks after the test, women who had heard nothing scored 45.9 on the anxiety scale. Those who had been told that the results were negative were still relatively anxious, but a bit less so at 42.4.

Prenatal diagnosis also raises the fear that medical attention will be diverted from treatment, from caring for the handicapped and from research to find the underlying causes. No longer are paediatric wards in New York filled with children with Tay-Sachs disease, Rothman says, because most couples at risk are aborting affected fetuses. The result, she says, is 'privatisation' of the tragedy of genetic disease. Abortion does not become an interim solution on the road to effective treatment and cure, because 'if the loss goes unrecognised, turned around into a solution, then the pressure is off'. This may well be a real danger, especially as government funds for biomedical research grow scarcer. Certainly, there has already been more interest in studying the fashionable molecular aspects of sickle cell anaemia than in the disease in patients. Hence we know little about why the disease develops so differently under different conditions, with some people much more severely affected than others.[28] Partly, this may also reflect institutionalised racism: research in Britain into the cause and treatment of cystic fibrosis, a disease mainly of white northern European communities, receives about 40 times more funding than does research into sickle cell anaemia (a disease mainly of the Afro-Caribbean communities).[29]

Yet prenatal diagnosis does not inevitably distort the direction of biomedical research, or provisions for treatment and support for people with genetic diseases. Ed Yoxen draws a helpful analogy with polio.[30] Since the development of a vaccine against the disease in the 1950s, the number of children afflicted has dropped markedly. Fewer people know of anyone with the disease, and medical authorities may feel obliged to support educational campaigns to encourage people to vaccinate their children. 'Surely no one would argue that we should abandon vaccination, either to remind ourselves what polio is like or to stiffen our resolve to care for future cases?' The same is true of genetic diseases, he argues: 'Prevention can lead to indifference, but this is not a valid argument for not trying to prevent the birth of children with genetic disease. It is an argument for working to prevent indifference . . .'. One safeguard may be to insist that genetic screening and treatment are combined in special units, as in thalassaemia and haemophilia centres in Britain. Furthermore, although it often sounds like special pleading on the part of molecular biologists, it must be true that research at the level of DNA does not lead only to the ability to screen prenatally for genetic disease. Such research should ultimately discover the defective proteins underlying specific genetic diseases, which are mostly unknown, and so lead to the possibility of finding a more effective treatment or cure. This is why charities devoted to various genetic diseases now fund much basic research – the worrying development is that in Britain at least charities now spend more money than the government does in supporting such research.

Rothman, along with some campaigners for disability rights, argues that prenatal diagnosis increases the social stigma of disability, too. Taking the pressure off society to care for less able members can lead to even less material and social support for disabled people. If a woman refuses to have the test, or refuses to abort an affected fetus, society may judge that it is she who is to 'blame' for bringing a handicapped child into the world, says Rothman. With little social support for women with less than 'normal' children, women are often forced to choose abortion, she says. Rothman also argues that if you choose not to abort, the early knowledge of a defect adds nothing but anguish to the rest of the pregnancy. But some groups for disability rights support the notion of screening because if a family has decided to go on, with the knowledge of what it will entail, they may be more committed to the infant, and make better parents.

At the root of much condemnation of prenatal screening is the notion that it is aimed at creating 'perfect' babies. Opinions differ about who supposedly wants such perfection: is it women, coerced by society, doctors, driven to excess by ambition and power, or even governments, in search of a 'master race'? For instance, a leading obstetrician in London, Charles Rodeck, argues that as families become smaller, attitudes to children have changed, creating an increased 'consumer demand' for perfect children.[31] Rothman speaks of 'technology-driven changes in standards'. The invention of the washing machine, she says, increased our standards of cleanliness. 'With new reproductive technology, will our standards for our children rise?' she asks. Still others argue that the quality control of prenatal screening is forced on women by the medical profession. At a conference on screening for genetic diseases organised by the King's Fund in London in 1987, Macintyre said, for instance, 'It is not true that women want perfect babies – doctors do.'

There is an element of truth in all these perspectives. In the short term, however, and given the enormous constraints on women, feminists must work to increase the choices offered to women, to make up their own minds with the best possible information, about how to run their own lives. Such a naively liberal argument acquires teeth if we look towards improving the social resources that would enhance freedom to choose. Access to information and unbiased counselling for women, now abysmally limited, is a central issue. So too is the wherewithal from government to support those affected by genetic disease.

Communication between 'expert' and 'patient' is notoriously inadequate, but is nowhere worse than in prenatal diagnosis. Macintyre points out, for instance, that some women do not really understand that prenatal tests will not enable doctors to treat an affected fetus. Doctors sometimes say that they can 'prevent' the baby being affected, and ensure that your baby is not ill. But this statement is ambiguous; doctors do not mean that they can 'cure' an affected child, or prevent the fetus from being affected by some disease: they can only abort an affected fetus and so 'prevent' the baby. Furthermore, says Macintyre, people often misinterpret information that is supposedly widely known, and need more information; for instance, many people think younger women are not at risk for Down's syndrome – the difference between relative risk (individually higher for older women) and attributed risk (most babies with Down's syndrome are born to younger women).

'Genetic counselling' thus becomes a central issue for feminists.[32] Feminists need to campaign vigorously in this field, to influence how a woman is given information, what she is told, and by whom. The term is a catch-all for attempts to give individuals information about their genetic status and the risks of passing on a particular genetic disease to a child.[33] In Britain, doctors dominate genetic counselling, with disastrous results. They are usually 'too busy', patronising and downright ignorant of the social and psychological consequences of genetic disease to provide clear and undirected information. Particularly in the US, a growing band of professional genetic counsellors are becoming influential. They argue that a counsellor should provide information on the meaning of the tests, the nature of the disease and so on, and then support the woman in her choice, whether she aborts the fetus or not. The counsellor should never give advice or colour a woman's decision. Yet such ideals are extremely difficult to achieve in practice. The product often of postgraduate courses in genetic counselling, they will find it difficult to avoid a 'medical' approach. Even if they attempt to provide a different perspective, they may well be overruled, as paramedical staff, by the doctor's higher status. Many counsellors are women, but they are still often far removed from their 'clients' in status, class, education and race or ethnic origins. And, as feminists such as Anne Finger[34] have pointed out, even counsellors have distinct stereotypes about disabilities and no claim to specialised knowledge of what it is like to grow up disabled or care for such a child.

The 'medicalisation' of social and ethical questions is a real danger. As Macintyre says, 'What it is like to have a child with the condition is better answered by support groups – doctors or midwives are not likely to know.' Similarly, self-help groups may be the best help for women who decide to abort an affected fetus. One such group in London, Support After Termination for Abnormalities (SATFA) offers information, counselling and support long after a woman leaves the hospital or clinic.[35] Government funding for such support groups, to which state health agencies could refer women, may be a promising approach.

Various bioethics committees set up by government or the medical establishment have now drawn up guidelines to govern prenatal testing and counselling. Most stress that all information discovered about the fetus must be disclosed to the woman screened. The information must be backed up with genetic counselling. Before any screening begins, which should be voluntary and confidential, there must be an intense educational campaign in the community.[36] Nonetheless, the issue of 'information' remains contentious. Rothman argues, for instance, that women may be ill equipped to cope with ambiguous diagnoses, of abnormalities of the sex chromosomes, say, that may have unknown outcomes for the child (see box 7.3). A woman must be given the right of 'informed refusal', says Rothman – the right to decide which things she wants to know about.

Knowledge of the sex of a child before birth is also a minefield. Will women abort fetuses because they are the 'wrong' sex? Already, the abortion of 'normal' female fetuses after amniocentesis is widespread in India, where the dowry system makes female children an expensive proposition.[37] Who is to decide whether to prevent such practices? A policy of making all information available to the woman is preferable, many feel, to relying on the 'discretions' of the doctor. Already there is often pressure on a woman to abort an affected fetus, or even to agree to an abortion before doctors will agree to perform an amniocentesis. Most commentators condemn this practice; as Macintyre says, it is important to allow women to have the test and then decide what to do, because it is difficult to know how one will behave in a hypothetical situation.

But perhaps women themselves will 'abuse' prenatal diagnosis, aborting fetuses for 'trivial' reasons. Rothman argues that chorionic villus sampling will only make matters worse. If it is easier to abort earlier, it becomes easier to abort for the wrong reasons, she argues, such as the sex of the child or a mild disability. What about Down's syndrome itself? Many people argue that these fetuses should not be aborted, as the children seem to lead happy, if foreshortened, lives. Who is to decide? 'Selective termination' implicitly judges the value or worth of a life, and the quality of that life. As treatment improves, as with cystic fibrosis and sickle cell disease, for instance, or our knowledge of other disorders such as

Down's syndrome increases, we need to reassess any judgements about the quality of those lives. Such considerations cannot be left to the medical profession; a doctor has no special knowledge of what it is like to be a person with Down's, for instance, or what it is like to care for that person. A woman who has already had a child with sickle cell disease, on the other hand, has considerable insights into the condition. Because it is women who are likely in our society to care for children, women are apt to consider carefully the nature of the child's life. No individual is better placed to make such a judgement.

'Science' is likely to be unhelpful in such decisions; it may even be unable to provide clearcut information on the physical consequences of a particular genetic lesion. It is often difficult to tell how severely an infant would be affected by looking at its DNA. Various diseases that are similar at the genetic level, such as forms of thalassaemia, produce symptoms that range from mild to severe. Some clinicians fail to distinguish between them, and pursue a blanket policy of termination for any fetus with a lesion in its haemoglobin genes. Similarly, mutations of two collagen genes that cause a bone disease called osteogenesis imperfecta can result in a bewildering array of symptoms, ranging from a fatal collapse of a baby's ribs at its first breath to a condition so mild that the tendency to break bones is hardly noticeable.[38]

Diseases that do not appear until adulthood present special problems too. Huntington's disease can now be diagnosed prenatally, with an accuracy of about 95 per cent in informative families. People carrying the gene for the disease invariably start to become demented in their forties, and suffer progressive degeneration of their nervous system. 'Presymptomatic tests' for adults at risk of having inherited the gene are now available, if the whole family across several generations co-operates and gives blood samples. Knowing whether you will be struck down in middle age has left people either 'with a profound feeling of relief' or 'shocked by the outcome, with intermittent depression', say researchers.[39]

Finally there are the 'psychiatric' disorders. Researchers have claimed to find a single gene that predisposes individuals to disorders such as manic depressive disease, but apparently not everyone who has the gene becomes a manic-depressive.[40] Molecular geneticists are eagerly searching for genes underlying schizophrenia and Alzheimer's disease as well. What anyone should do with such information is still a matter of much debate.

A leading doctor in thalassaemia screening in Britain, Bernadette Modell, argues that in the end we must leave all such decisions to the individual woman, for we make our best ethical choices when the course of our own lives is at stake.[41] Psychologists have documented our tendency to underrate the moral richness of other people's lives – we often think it likely that other people will make unethical decisions, but not ourselves. This myopia may be inevitable, as we live inside our own moral world, and best understand the complexity of the decisions we make ourselves. But we cannot improve on ethical decisions about abortion, as a whole, or prenatal diagnosis, by imposing laws on individuals, Modell argues. The only right way to influence individual choice is through changes in the social context in which a woman makes her decision by, say, providing support for disabled children.

That said, we still do not know what the implications for society will be if genetic screening becomes truly widespread and we may in the future want to ban certain practices, such as the abortion of fetuses on the basis of sex. Insurance companies are already discriminating against the victims of AIDS, or even people (single men) deemed to be a 'higher risk'. They would probably attempt to do the same in genetic screening, discriminating against someone with a genetic predisposition to, say, heart disease. Government legislation would be needed to make this illegal.

We might also understandably worry about the development of a 'eugenic' drive, based on some criterion imposed by the government of what is 'normal'. But a more genuine danger is not a drive to recreate the racial hygiene movement of the early years of this century, but, as Edward Yoxen puts it, a temptation 'to deprive people of some of their autonomy, in the belief that one acts for their own good. What lives on is perhaps not eugenics, but a kind of genetic paternalism.'[42] We can also gain some comfort from the abysmal track record of screening programmes that have adopted the 'top down' approach. Attempts to set up screening programmes for various minority groups work well and can enhance women's autonomy if the initiative comes from the local community, and is backed by a proper educational campaign. For instance, screening for thalassaemia in several Mediterranean countries gained ground with the support of the Church (see box 7.6). Screening for Tay-Sachs in the Jewish population of Washington and Baltimore took off after local rabbis endorsed the scheme. But in the early 1970s the US government's attempt to set up sickle cell screening was a disaster, despite heavy federal support. The black people of the US were summarily told that they were suffering from a neglected disorder, and offered screening without genetic counselling. Several states even made screening mandatory. The campaign created discrimination against blacks in jobs and health insurance, and fuelled racism.

In practice, doctors now make the choices for us, or at least set the questions we are asked. We have yet to see a revolution in genetic screening in the antenatal clinics largely because doctors are slow to take an interest in genetic tests and inform their patients of what is available. A recent survey of screening for Down's syndrome, in women over thirty-five in the west of Scotland, is a good example.[43] Despite a well-organised system, the programme reduced the incidence of Down's by only 5 to 8 per cent, although in theory the programme could achieve a fall of 35 per cent or more. A study in 1983 revealed the reasons. Women had moral or

Box 7.6. *Screening for Thalassaemia*

Thalassaemia is a good model for exploring the implications of prenatal diagnosis in practice, and presents, in many ways, a 'best case' scenario. For a start, the diseases are serious and widespread. About two hundred million people – 5 per cent of the world population – are carriers for the major inherited forms of anaemia, and at least 200,000 severely affected babies are born each year with thalassaemia or sickle cell disease. These are disorders of haemoglobin, the oxygen-carrying pigment in the blood. These diseases cause great suffering, particularly in Africa, the Indian sub-continent and the Mediterranean. In Thailand alone, with a population of 48 million, probably some 500,000 suffer some degree of chronic ill-health due to some form of thalassaemia. Several different forms are common – in the most severe, alpha thalassaemia, children die at birth. Children with the other common type, beta thalassaemia, need blood transfusions to stay alive and still suffer many damaging side effects.

The thalassaemias are not only common; they are also among the best studied single gene defects. A simple blood test can detect carriers – that is, those who have one defective gene and are at risk of producing an affected child if they reproduce with another carrier. A decade ago, researchers developed a technique of sampling fetal blood, through the umbilical cord, to enable prenatal diagnosis of the disorder, but the technique is risky and can be carried out only late in pregnancy. Prenatal diagnosis based on fetal DNA early in pregnancy is now possible.

The World Health Organisation (WHO) has for some years been supporting local projects designed to initiate widespread screening for thalassaemia in those countries most affected. Prenatal diagnosis for thalassaemia is widely accepted in Catholic countries such as Sardinia and Italy; indeed, medical centres screen virtually everyone of marriageable age in many Mediterranean countries. But many Islamic countries refuse to set it up. In Thailand, the largely Buddhist population

(Continued overleaf)

seems to find it acceptable if diagnosis is early in pregnancy, with the emphasis on the mother's well-being.

Initially, there were widespread fears that people might refuse to marry carriers, or that carriers would be socially stigmatised at work and so on. In fact, this did not happen. In Cyprus, where 1 in 35 marriages is at risk of producing an infant with severe thalassaemia, there was no change in the pattern of marriages. Carriers who married with one another merely then sought prenatal diagnosis. The authorities attribute the success of the project, even in a heavily Catholic country, to a huge education campaign that stressed the prevalence of the gene in the population and the evolutionary reason – that it conferred resistance to malaria.

Sardinia and Cyprus now have thriving programmes. Italy and Greece also have screening schemes, but the big mainland populations are more difficult to work with, because several different genetic mutations underlie the disease there. This makes it harder to set up simple DNA tests for carrier status or prenatal diagnosis. In Thailand, a battery of gene probes are needed to cover all the different mutations in the population. The tests are not yet sufficiently cheap and easy to use in small rural laboratories, restricting screening to hospitals in the cities. Yet the human cost of the disease is probably at its worst in Thailand, according to David Weatherall, of the John Radcliffe Hospital in Oxford. Either no treatment is available for affected children, or it is expensive. Families have been made financially destitute and healthy children starved as money goes to treat the afflicted child.

Things are better in Britain, where the NHS pays for treatment. But couples who have had an affected child often seek prenatal diagnosis, to prevent the distress of seeing another child afflicted with the gruelling treatments, or else they stop having children. Studies in Britain and Australia suggest that before prenatal diagnosis for thalassaemia was available, most couples at risk responded by stopping having children. In response to demand from the Cypriot community in London, Bernadette Modell of the University College Hospital has set up a thalassaemia screening programme in

London. With the help of Cypriot health workers and community groups, she has established a successful, sought-after service. A similar centre is at work in Oxford. Asian families in Britain have so far been much less interested in prenatal diagnosis for thalassaemia, however, perhaps through lack of communication at a grass roots level. In practice, the politics of voluntary screening programmes, and even some mandatory ones, have so far determined their success or failure: those imposed on a community at risk from above have failed.

In theory, every pregnant woman in Britain could be screened for carrier status for one form, beta thalassaemia, from the blood sample given at the first prenatal visit. Carriers have small red blood cells and low levels of haemoglobin. The hospital could then test the partner, and, if they were both carriers, they could be referred to genetic counsellors and offered prenatal diagnosis. Tests of fetal DNA, extracted either by CVS or amniocentesis, can give an answer 80 to 90 per cent of the time. Where DNA analysis fails to give a diagnosis, doctors can sample fetal blood from the umbilical cord, in the second trimester of pregnancy. But this ideal scenario, from a medical genetics point of view, rarely happens in practice. 'Ignorance about genetic disease and counselling is still widespread throughout the medical profession,' says Weatherall.

Thalassaemia remains the best example of how genetic screening and prenatal diagnosis can work. It is possible to detect carriers through a simple blood test, before they have had an affected child, and to test the fetus through accurate DNA tests. The disease is common enough in various countries (or among many identifiable immigrant groups in Britain) to make such screening feasible. Furthermore, it is easy for clinicians to justify screening even in crude monetary terms. In Cyprus, for example, the annual cost of the thalassaemia programme is equal to the cost of treating its existing 605 patients for five years. In Britain, the entire service could run for a year for less than the cost of treating a single patient for twenty years. In 1983 the WHO working party on prenatal diagnosis wholeheartedly concluded that prenatal diagnosis of thalassaemia and sickle cell is cost effective where the diseases are relatively common.

religious objections to the termination of pregnancy in 7 per cent of cases, and went to the clinic too late in pregnancy 16 per cent of the time. But in 50 per cent of the cases, the obstetrician failed to offer the woman amniocentesis. David Weatherall of the John Radcliffe Hospital in Oxford stresses the need for widespread education of the medical profession: 'Otherwise, we will end up with a powerful technology in the hands of a few specialised centres, not being fully used, and not benefiting most patients. This is already happening. I fear that there may be a long delay between what is possible in the research or reference laboratory and what patients are offered in the community.'[44]

Summary and Predictions

The speed of developments in molecular genetics is awesome, so it is impossible to predict the future with much certainty. Many commercial interests, from small biotechnology companies to large multinationals, are now investing in genetic diagnosis. The US Food and Drug Administration has not yet approved any devices or kits based on DNA probes to diagnose genetic diseases, but already there are rows over who owns gene probes and whether they can be patented. Much interest focuses on replacing the radioactive labels on probes with fluorescent ones, to make DNA tests cheaper and quicker. 'DNA fingerprinting' can now identify individuals by the pattern of various repeated regions of their DNA, and pinpoint their relatives. A new technique of amplifying DNA to make many copies of a single gene means that researchers need fewer cells to do DNA tests. Geneticists can now fingerprint amplified DNA from a single hair, or a drop of blood or semen. Forensic science is already transformed.

It is easy to conclude from all this that society will soon slide down one or other of several slippery slopes. 'To many, eliminating genetic defects sounds like a worthy goal. But we must realise that the category "genetic defect" is one capable of infinite expansion,' says Gena Corea and her colleagues.[45] But can't we in fact draw a line? That is the standard solution to a slippery slope. Advances in molecular genetics could lead to horrific social changes, but they need not. As Yoxen says, a slippery slope argument is 'wrongheaded, very conservative, even reactionary, because it says so little about what we ought to do.'[46]

In any case, the nature of genetic disease makes an organised conspiracy to create 'a more perfect human race' unlikely. Cost alone makes it difficult to imagine that any government would launch a programme to screen all pregnant women for a handful of genetic diseases, let alone the population at large. After all, doctors in Britain could routinely screen all pregnant women for diseases such as sickle cell disease or thalassaemia, but screening is in fact sporadic and patchy.[47] In Britain today, at any rate, the risk of an imposed screening programme seems small; in fact, people at risk of passing on sickle cell disease have long lobbied Parliament for better provision for both treatment and screening. Screening newborns for the disease could be done cheaply, through a simple blood test, and would enable the children to be better protected against infection, the biggest danger for them. Not unreasonably, many have concluded that the government ignores the disease because it affects mostly black people. In Britain 5,000 people suffer from the disease – as many as from haemophilia A – yet the facilities for screening and treatment resemble the situation for haemophilia of twenty to thirty years ago.

It is worth remembering too, when we extrapolate into the future, that just as all women are not the same, neither are all genetic diseases. Many of the diseases carried on the X-chromosome, for example, arise from new mutations – as many as a third of the cases of Duchenne muscular dystrophy, for instance. In these cases, no family history of the disease alerts a couple to seek prenatal diagnosis. Screening every pregnant woman for the disease would be prohibitively expensive, as well as dangerous. So in the case of Duchenne, prenatal diagnosis really helps only to prevent the birth of afflicted sons to mothers known to be carriers because they have already had a boy with DMD. This is hardly the stuff of a eugenic programme.

Nor are the screening programmes we now have all that 'effective' in diagnosing other fetal abnormalities. Chromosomal abnormalities such as Down's are more common throughout the world than single-gene defects. But present programmes that focus on individual women at highest risk miss most of the affected fetuses – again, not a very promising result for a eugenic scheme. One might argue that chorionic villus sampling, because it is performed earlier when an abortion is less traumatic, might lead doctors to lower the age limit. Younger women might then be encouraged to undergo tests for Down's. But again, the cost of prenatal tests is high, and no machine can yet analyse the chromosomes of a cell as well as the experienced human eye (although some devices, such as fluorescent cell sorters, now come close).

The ultimate in prenatal diagnosis – detecting genetic disease in an embryo, before it has implanted in the womb – is now feasible.[48] There are various ways of going about this, which seem feasible in theory. Embryologists could screen young embryos created through IVF at several ages. At the two-cell stage, researchers have successfully split mouse embryos in two, and frozen one half while awaiting the results of genetic tests on the other half. Research on monkeys has shown that it is possible to 'biopsy' an older embryo, by clipping off a few cells of the 'trophoblast' which will go on to form the placenta. Researchers have now shown that with human embryos it is possible to remove one cell at the six-cell stage, and test that cell for the presence of a particular gene, without damaging the rest of the embryo.

Why go to all this effort? The idea is that many couples known to be at risk of passing on a severe genetic disease would want to have their embryos screened. A couple wanting children could thus avoid the trauma of repeated abortions of affected fetuses, detected later in pregnancy through chorionic villus sampling or amniocentesis. The UK Thalassaemia Society, in its submission to the Warnock Committee in the early 1980s, said that the ideal would be to be able to start a pregnancy knowing from the time of implantation that the fetus would be unaffected.

There are several stumbling blocks to this goal, however. At the moment, the technique of chorionic villus sampling causes less inconvenience and discomfort to the mother than the removal of eggs for IVF, and is less expensive. Furthermore, IVF and embryo transfer has such a low success rate that it might take several atttempts to achieve a pregnancy (although success rates might be higher for fertile couples). As Yoxen puts it, it would be a matter of exchanging 'the uncertainty in an established pregnancy for uncertainty about whether a pregnancy will be established. It is not obvious that this is an improvement.'[49] The risk of an affected child from parents who were both carriers could far more simply be avoided by artificial insemination by a donor – although the husband would then not be the genetic father.

Despite these difficulties for the idea of 'preimplantation diagnosis' many fear that the screening of embryos will become widespread and lead to the ultimate obsession with 'perfection'. Jacques Testard, a leading IVF specialist in France, has publicly withdrawn from such research, for fear, he says, that soon everyone will want to have their babies by IVF, in the belief that this will ensure that they have a perfect baby.[50] The feminist biologist Ruth Hubbard, of Harvard University, can also easily imagine a future in which IVF is the norm: 'At that point, "in body fertilisation" will not only have come to seem old-fashioned and quaint, but downright foolhardy, unhealthy and unsafe.'[51]

It is impossible to say that this cannot happen. But it would be enormously expensive to produce all babies through IVF and difficult to prevent people from reverting to normal means. It would be far cheaper for a government to launch a eugenic drive along Nazi lines, by simply killing people or imprisoning them. Why not practise infanticide, destroying affected babies cheaply at birth, rather than risk damaging an unaffected fetus through costly diagnostic procedures?

The final futuristic scenario is that of 'gene therapy'.[52] The idea of replacing a defective gene in an adult is not all that different from organ transplants or blood transfusions. Several research teams in the US have nearly perfected ways of introducing genes into bone marrow cells to correct various deficiencies in blood cells. It might be possible to treat thalassaemia in this way relatively soon. This kind of gene therapy, called somatic gene therapy, seems to offer few, if any, new ethical dilemmas. It is much like a bone marrow transplant, say, for people suffering from leukaemia, except that in this case the patients would receive their own cells back again, with a gene added. In experiments on animals a modified virus successfully carries a gene into these cells, correcting thalassaemia. This approach could develop into an effective treatment for children born with serious genetic diseases. It could also provide an alternative for those people with a conscientious objection to abortion. Yet it will probably remain a medically risky and uncertain treatment for years to come. Careful controlled clinical trials, with full and informed consent, must temper the enthusiasm of doctors and scientists working in the field and control their ambition to be 'first'.

The notion of 'germline gene therapy' – introducing genes into a fertilised egg to alter its genetic characteristics and that of its offspring – is more frightening. This kind of genetic alteration would affect all the cells in the organism, and be passed on to its offspring. It is now possible to introduce new genes into the single-cell embryos of mice, rats, or even sheep and pigs. The result is called a 'transgenic' animal because a new gene has been transferred into it. Researchers usually inject the single-celled embryo with many copies of a particular gene and sometimes one or more copies end up incorporated into the genetic material of the cell. As a result, the adult animal ends up with the introduced gene present in all its cells, including the germ cells that make sperm or egg. This technique could conceivably one day be applied to human embryos, to cure diseases caused by defective genes or even to introduce new characteristics. It would be valuable particularly for those diseases such as cystic fibrosis where affected infants are already damaged at birth.

Yet germline gene therapy is a distant prospect, not just for ethical reasons. It is a hit-or-miss affair in laboratory animals at the moment. Most of the animal embryos do not take up the foreign DNA. Some of those do die before completing development, or suffer severe defects of one kind or another caused by the random insertion of the foreign genes into its genetic material. There is even the risk that the genetic damage may later lead to the development of cancer. Finally the gene has to work normally once in place, and such fine control is difficult to achieve.

After very many attempts, researchers have produced mice that grow bigger because they have a gene for growth hormone from rats. In Edinburgh, researchers have produced transgenic sheep that produce in their milk a human protein, a blood clotting factor given to people with haemophilia.[53] The idea is that we might be able to produce livestock that secrete useful proteins for industry or medicine in their milk. A strain of transgenic pigs given growth hormone genes do not grow bigger, but seem to produce leaner muscles. But when it comes to treating human diseases it would be much easier to carry out preimplantation diagnosis and weed out defective embryos.

Despite commercial pressures from agriculture to develop the techniques for producing transgenic animals, it should be possible to block a 'slippery slope' moving from somatic gene therapy to germline therapy in humans. Virtually all researchers condemn the notion of applying the procedure to human embryos, given the risks of some unknown complication resulting from genetic intervention. Furthermore, the alternatives – somatic gene therapy, prenatal diagnosis or preimplantation diagnosis – are further advanced and inherently simpler. The religious right might prefer gene therapy on embryos to prenatal genetic screening leading to abortion; and their support for 'therapy' might form part of the move towards a total abolition of abortion. But to develop the technique, the anti-abortionists would have to allow research on human embryos and the discarding of faulty ones, which most conservatives oppose.

Huxley's famous novel concentrated on the horrors created by a centralised state, but today we have more to fear from the commercialisation of human genetics. As Yoxen puts it: 'The excesses of the in vitro fertilisation business, the surrogacy industry and the market in sex predetermination services all arise because parents' anxieties are perceived as profit opportunities by people with a skill to sell.'[54] The solution to such excesses as 'designer children', if indeed they ever become possible, is then the control of the genetic entrepreneurs. Legislation to outlaw such services, as has been done for commercial surrogacy in Britain, is one effective approach.

But we must also work to alter the social and economic context in which women bear and rear children, to enhance the autonomy of women. 'An obsession with eliminating so-called 'defects' from the human population in a search for a more perfect human race could lead to an increasing intolerance for those of us who are physically challenged and a reduction in the already meagre social support services for us,' feminists point out.[55] This is certainly a possible consequence of prenatal screening, but it is one that has to be fought directly, rather than through a wholesale rejection of prenatal diagnosis. As Yoxen says, we must work to broaden and deepen the extent of 'environmental change' that provides support to disabled people. The notion of changing diet or wearing spectacles or hearing aids, is a widely accepted solution to some perceived disability. But less individualistic solutions, and often more expensive ones, meet more resistance. Writes Yoxen: 'We tend not to devote the considerable resources required to make the physical environment less challenging for people with spina bifida, who are likely to suffer from a degree of spasticity. Every intrinsic deficiency is linked to an "implicit environment" that sets limits on what we are prepared to change. It follows,' he argues, 'that what we classify as a disease is a convention, dependent partly on our technology.'[56]

Part 3

8. Towards a Reproductive Future?

Prenatal diagnosis and the possibility of germline gene therapy invoke the spectre of a future in which 'perfect' children are made to order. Other possible developments, however, could also lend themselves to such eugenic ends. Ectogenesis, cloning and parthenogenesis are all possible forms of reproductive technology that could, some critics argue, enhance patriarchal control of reproduction, and allow greater control over the 'quality' of babies produced. These possibilities – particularly ectogenesis – provoke fears both of Machiavellian scientists creating a new social order and of a total takeover of women's reproductive role. It is just those fears that have led to the call for a total resistance to reproductive technologies.

Yet these possibilities are just that: possibilities. None of them is yet fact, and the problems they raise for women and for feminism may well be quite different from those raised, say, by the use of in vitro techniques. If we are going to consider them as possibilities for the future, then we have to try to assess how likely they are to become reality: only then can we work out their impact on women's lives. In this chapter, we consider the future in two ways. First, we examine the likelihood of those forms of technology that evoke most anxiety – such as ectogenesis – and consider whether, if such technologies were to exist, they would substantially alter women's lives. In the second part, we look at scenarios of the future described by some feminist critics of reproductive technologies.

Ectogenesis

Ectogenesis means the creation of life wholly outside the human body. In practice, this would mean the production of babies in carefully controlled and monitored laboratory conditions. Some feminists, such as Simone de Beauvoir and Shulamith Firestone, have argued that one reason for women's subordination is that they are handicapped by the necessity to give birth. Pregnancy and birth, they suggested, inevitably restrict what women can do, and patriarchy has taken advantage of that. That restriction, Firestone believed, could be lifted if we had access to ectogenesis, if we could take 'barbaric' pregnancies out of the bodies of women and free them for other pursuits. There could be other advantages, too: widespread use of ectogenesis might reduce the need for surrogacy, as 'infertility' would be much less of a social problem for women.

Ectogenesis could be defended on moral grounds if it could be shown to provide social benefits. In their book *The Reproduction Revolution*, Peter Singer and Deanne Wells[1] describe a number of possible benefits that might result from widespread acceptance of ectogenesis. Some of these seem, on the face of it, to be benefits that feminists would accept. Consider, for instance, their suggestion that ectogenesis could eliminate or reduce the need for surrogacy. Feminists have certainly had much to worry about with surrogacy, so the notion that ectogenesis could provide an alternative way for infertile people to have children seems attractive.

Yet many of the problems remain. Ectogenesis is likely to be costly. If it was available, it would remain either in private health care, and so be available only to the rich, or it would be a scarce resource within a state-funded system of health care. In the latter case, it would probably be like IVF now –

available only to those who are selected by various screening criteria.

Justifying the provision of ectogenesis on the grounds of avoiding surrogacy also assumes that it is morally acceptable to insist that people have their 'own' genetic children. But why should it be acceptable? As we noted in Chapter One, the insistence on genetic relatedness to our children reduces women's involvement with bearing children to that of men's, and devalues the role of social parenting. There is, one critic argued, no clear moral reason why we should justifiably ensure *genetic* continuity: 'If the desires of the childless are a legitimate reason for the state to act to provide them with children to nurture, then adoption of unwanted children is preferable to ectogenesis in doing so.'[2]

Another argument put forward by Singer and Wells is that ectogenesis could reconcile the conflict between anti-abortionists and feminists' demand for a woman's right to choose. Unwanted fetuses, they argue, could be put into artificial wombs for later adoption (although this is clearly in conflict with the emphasis on genetic continuity). But is the conflict really reconciled? There are two reasons for feminists to be suspicious of this justification of ectogenesis. First, if the fetus is to be removed uninjured from the womb, it would have to be fairly well developed: at present, early abortions involve fetal destruction. That would mean that the pregnant woman has to wait until mid-pregnancy, and may then have to have either an induction or a caesarian delivery. Second, a woman bearing an unwanted pregnancy may not want to hand over her fetus to an artificial womb. Just as most women, given the choice, would prefer to end the pregnancy by abortion than to hand over a child at term for adoption, so most women would probably prefer early abortion to the idea of transferring an older fetus to a technological incubator.

Ectogenesis, then, might be less liberating for women than Firestone believed. More recent feminist writing has taken quite different views of women's role in reproduction. Rather than viewing women as inevitably limited by pregnancies, feminists now tend to celebrate women's unique biological role. They have also emphasised that the arrival of ectogenesis could be liberating only if we had a world in which women were truly equal. And if we were truly equal, then women's biological processes would not be despised, thus reducing any demand to take pregnancy out of women's bodies. But in any other world, ectogenesis would surely be oppressive.

Feminists may have reason to fear the motives of men who advocate ectogenesis; it is certainly possible that some of them desire to have ultimate control over reproduction. Robyn Rowland pointed out that, 'Researchers need only to find an artificial environment which would bridge the gap from fourteen days to twenty-four weeks' of gestation, and they would have total control over reproduction.[3] If that were possible, then reproduction could indeed be taken out of women's wombs. So far, control is possible only at either end: in the case of early embryos and fetuses old enough to be able to survive independently in incubators. But that does not make total technological control of gestation a reality. For the time being, at least, ectogenesis remains unfeasible.

Most biologists believe that there is no intrinsic reason why it should be *impossible*; there is no basic biological reason why development could not take place outside the uterus of which we are aware. Why, then, does the reality remain so far off? One reason is that we are still in abysmal ignorance about the detailed processes of interaction between the mother's body and the fetus. The interaction is so subtle that it may be extremely difficult to mimic with accuracy.

The practical and biological difficulties associated with ectogenesis may well remain huge. Critics invoke an image of 'babies in bottles', surrounded by some sort of appropriate fluid medium, maintained at constant temperature. Would that the biology of pregnancy were that simple! The fluid surrounding a fetus is not static; both the fetal and maternal bodies are constantly changing it. So ectogenesis would have to mimic that continuous dynamic change; it would also have to mimic accurately the dramatic changes occurring at birth. The act of birth (whether caesarian or vaginal) brings about all kinds of changes to fetal physiology. Taking air into the lungs for the first time, for instance, provokes changes in the way that blood is pumped through the heart. We simply do not know yet how that process would take place if fetuses were grown entirely in bottles and then removed. We are nowhere near having the expertise to do all of these things outside of women's bodies, and we may never be able to mimic pregnancy completely.

The possibility of taking pregnancies to term outside the uterus is rather nearer for laboratory mice than it is for women. Mice have short pregnancies, and the fetuses depend on a placenta for a relatively shorter period (all fetuses gain nourishment initially from a simple yolk sac, before the placenta is fully functional; fetal mice depend on the yolk sac for a longer proportion of the pregnancy). So, the kind of technique that is required to maintain the human embryos for fourteen days is sufficient to maintain a mouse embryo for half of its gestation. Some biologists feel that, even if taking a mouse embryo to term outside the womb is difficult, we may still gain much useful knowledge in the process. Anne McLaren, a leading British embryologist, suggests that 'The knowledge gained . . . would certainly advance our understanding of the causes of birth defects, and the interactions between mother and implanted embryo in a normal pregnancy.' But, she goes on, 'to adapt such technology from the mouse to a species such as our own, with a large fetus and a protracted gestation period, would be a colossal task. At present there seems no reason to think it would ever be attempted; even if vast resources were to be devoted to it, the chances of achieving a successful result before the end of the twenty-first century would be slim.'[4]

They are slim indeed. However malevolent patriarchy may seem at times, it is unlikely to encourage total or widespread use of ectogenesis unless it was cost-effective and easily controlled. As McLaren argues, it is likely to be hugely expensive, somewhat akin to the costs of keeping someone in intensive care for many months (at least). So, even if it were available, it would be available only to a few.

Nor may ectogenesis be as easily controlled as women can be. We can, of course, readily envisage all kinds of unpleasant scenarios of the future, in which patriarchal societies have pursued their misogynist logic so that women's reproduction is completely controlled; and we can imagine how ectogenesis might become a part of that logic. But it is important to remember that the technology is not *necessary* to that logic. It is, moreover, unlikely to be used on a *global* scale, because of the cost. Men would always need women to produce the rest – and more cheaply, too.

By describing ectogenesis as merely 'closing the gap' between early embryos and fetuses capable of surviving independently, feminist critics are in danger of portraying the fetus in a similar way to those who oppose women's rights to abortion. Pregnancy consists of far more than isolated fetuses making their lonely way from fertilised eggs to premature baby units. It is more than just 'closing a gap' precisely *because* women's bodies are needed, too. So, while ectogenesis could, conceivably, be used in ways that intensify male power, it is unlikely both technologically, and in economic terms, in the foreseeable future.

Cloning

Cloning is perhaps a bit more feasible – although here, too, its feasibility and implications are often overstated. Strictly speaking, cloning is the production of a number of genetically identical individuals. The idea seems to invoke images of hordes of 'photocopy' people, and feminist critics often fear that it will be *men* – especially rich, powerful and unpleasant ones – who want to produce 'copies' of themselves through technology.

This fear rests on many assumptions. The first is that

genetic identity means complete identity. It does not, as anyone who has paid any attention to nature's experiments with cloning will tell you. Monozygotic twins (that is, they are derived from one egg, and are 'identical') are genetically identical: yet they are usually far from being 'identical' as people. The genes we inherit can interact throughout development with their environment in a multitude of ways. Those who speculate what wonderful theories might be concocted by a clone of Einsteins might well be disappointed.

The second is that, at present, it is simply not possible to produce a new human individual as a result of 'copying' cells from an adult – as would be needed to make 'copies of Einstein'. What scientists *can* do, however, is to remove the nucleus from a fertilised egg – so removing the egg's genetic information – and replace it with a nucleus taken from a very young embryo. So, you could take nuclei from several cells in a single embryo and transplant them into fertilised eggs without nuclei, thus producing several genetically identical individuals. In mammals, such as mice, swapping nuclei between fertilised eggs has been done, so that an egg from one strain of mouse is given a nucleus from another strain.

Still, putting into an egg a nucleus from another egg or from a very early embryo is hardly 'copying' an adult person. The trouble is, it has proved impossible so far to get an egg to start developing if it is given a nucleus from an *adult* cell. Partly this is because most adult cells have become specialised during development (see box 8.1). Specialisation involves switching some genes off permanently, and switching others on: as a result, the genes are no longer capable of directing the development of the *whole* organism. A liver cell is quite different from a heart cell, say, because it has different genes that are active. Partly, too, not all cells of the body contain exactly the same genes: scientists now believe that the genes we inherit at fertilisation can be further rearranged during cell development, so that some cells end up with slightly different genes than others (in mammals,

> **Box 8.1. *Why Clone Frogs?***
>
> Why should scientists want to take out a nucleus from a fertilised egg, and replace it with a nucleus from an older animal? The answer is that it allows them to study one of the most mysterious facts about early development: a newly fertilised egg is one cell, containing many genes. As it develops, it divides to form many cells and eventually to form many different *kinds* of cells – muscle cells, brain cells and so on. But once these different kinds have formed, they are incapable of changing to anything else: once a liver cell, always a liver cell, however many times it divides. So, an important difference is that, early on, the cells of the embryo have the potential to become *any* kind of cell in the body, but they lose that potential as development proceeds, even though they contain more or less exact copies of the genes. By inserting nuclei from older embryos, scientists can discover at what point the cells lose their potential to be generalists and become specialised.

some cells of the immune system do this, although scientists do not yet know if any other cells do).

In frogs, the subject of most of the earlier experiments, scientists have had somewhat more luck in using nuclei from more developed individuals of the same species. They have, for instance, been able to get eggs to divide if the eggs are given nuclei obtained from the gut of a tadpole. But, again, they have failed to persuade eggs to divide and develop if they are given nuclei from an adult frog.

The biological message seems to be that once cells have differentiated into specific 'types' the genes they contain no longer work in the same way, and are no longer capable of imparting all the relevant information to direct the development of a whole adult animal from scratch. Even in frogs it is only tadpoles that retain some potential for imparting information: once they reach adulthood, that potential has been lost. But in mammals, including humans, that potential to translate information from genes into whole animals is lost almost immediately after fertilisation.

It may become feasible for scientists eventually to 'switch on' genes again later in development, long after they have been 'switched off' to become specialised cells. *If* they can learn to do that, then it may become possible to transplant nuclei from older, more differentiated, cells in cloning experiments. But that is a far cry from assuming that they will be able to make copies of adult men or women. By the time humans reach adulthood, some, at least, of their DNA may have changed by mutation. Most of these changes have no effect on our bodily function because most will occur in genes that have been switched off or are controlled by other genes (though some can eventually lead to cells becoming cancerous); but they could well prove disastrous if they were given free rein to develop without those controls in a pre-embryo.

That is not to say, though, that fears are entirely misplaced: what might be possible is that someone decides to produce several eggs, perhaps on an IVF programme, and then freezes them as an insurance for future generations. As it *is* possible to induce early development using nuclei from early embryos – at least in mice – it might become possible to use nuclei from early human embryos to create several genetically identical individuals. This may be possible, but there would be little point to transplanting nuclei in order to do it. Why not simply split the cells as soon as the fertilised egg divides into two? This is, after all, how nature creates clones in the form of twins. It is, moreover, a technique that has been used to create genetically identical twins in some species of domestic animals (such as sheep and cattle).

We do not yet know if there are limits to the number of times an early embryo can be divided in this way; perhaps if you divide it too many times the cells will just die. Yet this is probably the only way in which the much-feared armies of genetically identical people *could* be created, at least in the foreseeable future. As Anne McLaren has pointed out, small numbers of genetically identical people have never been something we have worried about; we don't, after all, think we should kill one of a pair of twins. What frightens critics is not one or two genetically identical individuals, but tens of hundreds, created deliberately to supply some dreadful social need.

There is one good biological reason why this might not be too good an idea, and that is precisely the genetic similarity of these armies. Should a new disease arise to which people with that set of genes are particularly vulnerable, they could all become infected. However good we become at medical control of disease, the story of AIDS should remind us that new diseases can arise over which we have little control. It would also be relatively easy to kill large numbers of genetically identical people using biological warfare; if the attacker finds a bacterium, say, that will kill one, then it will probably kill all of them. Genetically identical people will all have the same inherent strengths and weaknesses; with a new disease, they could all be wiped out.

Human-Animal Hybrids

Although the idea of creating human-animal hybrids fills most people with horror, it is equally unlikely that society would want to do so on any large scale. As with cloning, we have to ask for what purpose armies of weird creatures might be produced. The suggestion that the production of such hybrids might be morally justified because they could undertake unpleasant, menial jobs, thus freeing humans for more uplifting or interesting tasks[5] assumes, as we have argued, that producing a living thing for the purpose is cost effective. This seems unlikely.

Yet it is this possibility of half-human hybrids that seems closer: as hamster eggs are used to test for the viability of sperm (only properly shaped, motile sperm will be able to penetrate the outer layer, the zona pellucida, of the egg: this can be observed under the microscope as a means of assessing sperm: see box 8.2), fears have been expressed that 'mad scientists' might be creating hamster-human hybrids. This fear was, indeed, expressed in the report from the Warnock Committee, and the Government's draft White Paper (1987).

Hamster-human hybrids are not, in fact, likely to result from using hamster eggs in this way; they simply will not develop far enough. Still, it is possible that eggs from other species might develop considerably further, and the Warnock Committee accordingly recommended that such use of eggs from other species be subject to strict control so that they are destroyed after their use for testing the viability of sperm. The anti-abortion pressure group, SPUC, goes further, and recommends that all use of eggs from other species be banned.[6] At present, it seems unlikely that any such embryos would develop very far, and, even if they began to develop they might well be rejected by the mother's uterus (assuming that she had co-operated – or been coerced – with the transfer of such a hybrid).

Whether it would be morally acceptable to use human eggs or sperm to create half-human hybrids, it does not seem likely that society would ever condone the manufacture of such creatures on any significant scale. Even if there were societal controls, some unscrupulous scientists might be motivated by idle curiosity to see if it was possible. We may find this thoroughly distasteful, but creating a single hybrid does not, in itself, constitute a social threat. It would be the manufacture of hordes of such hybrids, or the coercion of women to bear such offspring that could do that.

Parthenogenesis

In principle, parthenogenesis – the creation of a human being only from an egg, without the participation of sperm – would be another way of creating individuals technologically. Parthenogenesis does occur naturally: it happens occasionally, for instance, in various kinds of lizards, and even in some

Box 8.2. *How Likely Are Animal-Human Hybrids?*

Hamster eggs fertilised as a test for the viability of human sperm do not develop: they divide once and then stop. Fertilisations sometimes occur between species in nature: and when they do, the product rarely develops very far. Species have evolved all kinds of elaborate mechanisms precisely to *prevent* interbreeding. Eggs, for instance, have very specific receptors on their surface membrane, to which only sperm from the same species can attach – if they get that far. Sperm from other species can usually reach the surface of the egg only if the outer layer, the zona, is not there – as in cases when it has been removed for a scientific experiment. In normal circumstances it will be there: even the hamster egg test for human sperm will work only if the zona has been removed first, and it works simply because the hamster egg is odd, in that it allows 'foreign' sperm through its surface. As far as apes are concerned (our closest relatives biologically), human sperm will get through the zona of eggs from gibbons, and possibly other apes: but that still does not mean they will necessarily fertilise, at least under normal conditions of fertilisation. Fertilisation itself is not merely a matter of sperm entering egg; it is a lengthy process that ends as the 'pronuclei' from egg and sperm fuse.

So scientists are not about to create strange mythical creatures that are half human and half hamster, say. For the moment at least, that is simply not biologically possible. There are, however, two ways in which scientists can produce offspring from two species. The first is by using a surrogate mother from one species for a fertilised egg of another species. This is possible only if the two species are sufficiently closely related – a horse has been used as a surrogate mother for a rare species of zebra, for example. The other method involves mixing up cells from early embryos of two species. This is sometimes done to breed endangered species, or to increase the productivity of agricultural animals. One way of doing this is simply to mix cells from the embryos of two species: goat and sheep embryos have been mixed, for instance, to

> make a strange animal looking like a bit of each. What to call this animal is causing some concern – a 'geep' is one possibility. This kind of animal made up of cells from embryos that are quite different genetically is called a chimera. Another kind of mixing involves mixing the inner embryonic cells that are destined to form the embryo of one species with cells destined to form the outer layers (and which would go to form part of the placenta) of another species. The resultant embryo will be genetically all one species – a sheep, for example – but can be carried by a surrogate of another species, such as a goat, if its outer layer consists of goat cells. The uterus of the surrogate animal will recognise these cells as being of the 'right' species and would not reject the embryo (as it normally would a sheep embryo). These 'mixed' animals are not the same as a hybrid made by fertilising an egg with a sperm from another species – for example, crossing a horse and a donkey to create a sterile mule.

birds, such as turkeys. But parthenogenetic individuals never survive pregnancy in mammals. Although it has proved possible in scientific experiments to induce early development parthenogenetically in mammal eggs (by mechanically or chemically stimulating them to divide) they always die not long after.

If it were possible, parthenogenesis in humans could, of course, be a virgin birth: but, unlike the well-known example, all such births would be female. They would usually contain only half the full number of chromosomes, as they would derive from the mother's egg alone. Or, these maternal chromosomes could divide to create a double set.

Scientists might also, in theory, be able to create a parthenogenetic embryo with the full number of chromosomes by fusing two eggs, much in the way that sperm and egg fuse in fertilisation. Such 'oval fusion', uniting two sets of genetic information is not, in theory, fundamentally different from any other form of fertilisation, even though the offspring would be just as 'artificially' created as any created by laboratory cloning.

Parthenogenesis of any kind has not generally raised feminist hackles. Creating female offspring is not something that we would associate with any intensification of patriarchy – and there is always the possibility of using parthenogenesis as a means of increasing *women's* control of reproduction: we could do it for ourselves. Men, too, have seen in this possibility the seeds of a 'redundant male', no longer necessary for reproduction.[7]

It is already possible for scientists to create 'fertilised' eggs with genes from two female parents, or from two male parents, at least in experiments with some animals. But, unfortunately for theories of redundant males, development in mammals stops unless the fertilised egg has one set of genes from a male and one from a female: it seems that certain genes that are essential for the formation of the tissues that develop into the fetal membranes and the placenta work properly only if they have been inherited from the father (see Chapter Six) – they are chemically altered in the formation of sperm. Likewise, certain genes that are essential for the early development of the fetus itself have to come from the mother, being specially 'processed' as her eggs are formed. So, although we get roughly half our genes at random from each parent, it seems to matter whether certain genes come from our mother or our father.

For some reason that scientists do not yet understand, something happens to these special genes during the formation of eggs and sperm. Not only is the number of chromosomes reduced to half, but the activity of some of the genes is altered chemically, depending upon whether they are inside a sperm or an egg.

A parthenogenetic embryo, artificially created, say, by the fusion of two eggs, does not contain genes that must come through the paternal line for normal development to proceed. The embryo would begin to develop normally, but lacks the necessary 'extra-embryonic' support system and so does not implant properly into the wall of the womb. An embryo created solely from paternal genes would also fail. It develops into a lump of tissue similar to membranes, but would lack the embryo-forming cells. Occasionally, though rarely, this happens in nature; an egg may be fertilised by two sperm, or the fertilising sperm may divide even before it can combine with the nucleus of the egg. The egg nucleus in either case seems to break down or be pushed out, and the cells begin to divide with genes derived only from the father. But without the special maternal genes, it cannot develop into an embryo: instead, it forms a lump of undifferentiated tissue. Medically, these are called hydatiform moles.

Perhaps some of the problems with techniques such as cloning and parthenogenesis will be overcome in the future. It is also possible that they will be insurmountable problems: we cannot be sure that we will ever find out completely what 'makes life tick'. Either way, they are not technologies that are imminent, however terrifying they can sometimes seem.

Earlier, we pointed to some different views of science and scientists that underpin debates on reproductive technologies. Many scientists themselves do see science as morally neutral, and capable of good, while seeing the need for some state control to limit its less desirable consequences. New developments could, in practice, offer women some advantages. Cloning and ectogenesis, for instance, could be techniques which might be used to overcome problems of infertility or genetic defect. There are, of course, ethical problems with doing so, and the cost implications are great; nevertheless, it remains feasible that these techniques *could* be used in ways that some people at least would consider beneficial. This kind of research has, moreover, yielded much information about how early embryos develop, which in turn has been medically useful.

To critics of reproductive technologies, though, it is ectogenesis and cloning which seem to invoke the greatest horror. From Leon Kass's suggestion that scientists are misled to the notion that they are in some way rather evil, no scientist who works on developing such techniques can, it seems, be trusted. For Kass, scientists are in danger of dehumanising reproduction in their belief that they can ultimately control nature;[8] for many feminist critics, the danger is that reproduction becomes defeminised. Worse, men might take it over completely. It is just that fear that we could move inevitably towards a world in which women were 'farmed' for their eggs, and in which men reproduced themselves through cloning and ectogenesis, that has motivated many feminists to reject reproductive technologies entirely.

Farming Women?

Gena Corea writes at length, and movingly, in *The Mother Machine*, of the uncaring attitudes displayed towards animals by the men who routinely practise egg harvesting as part of selective programmes of cattle breeding. She sees in this a parallel which women should heed: referring to companies with names like Embryo West and Portable Embryonics, she suggests that 'Perhaps within a few years firms with names such as these will be handling – not the eggs of cattle, but of women.'[9] Corea likens egg harvesting and the transfer of embryos in cattle, following Andrea Dworkin, to the creation of a 'reproductive brothel' which is fast becoming a possibility. 'While sexual prostitutes sell vagina, rectum and mouth', she says, 'reproductive-prostitutes will sell other body parts: womb; ovaries; eggs.'[10]

Using hormones to induce multiple ovulation is widely used in the American agriculture industry (and increasingly so in Britain) in order to breed larger numbers of offspring from prize cows. The cow is 'superovulated' with hormones, and then inseminated artificially, using previously frozen sperm. Two weeks later, any resulting embryos are flushed out (by means of catheters inserted into the womb) and are then put into an 'inferior' recipient cow. So, one prize cow could yield several embryos rather than one calf a year.

Corea pursues the analogy with cattle in creating a scenario of the 'reproductive brothel'. It is without doubt a chilling picture:

> In the brothel, on the appropriate days of their cycles, women would line up for Pergonal shots [one of the hormones that, at the time of Corea's writing, was most frequently used to induce ovulation] which will stimulate their ovaries. Engineers would superovulate only the top 10 to 20 per cent of the female population in the brothel. Then, after following the development of the eggs through ultrasound and blood tests, they would operate on the women to extract the eggs. Perhaps they would allow the women to heal from the operation every other month so that women would only be subjected to surgery six times a year.[11]

She goes on to speculate that ovaries might be removed from 'prize' women upon their death, to salvage eggs from the ovaries, 'perhaps by using enzymes to eat away the connective tissue and release hundreds of thousands of eggs . . . A woman could be used for reproduction long after she is dead.' Alternatively, women who were never born could be so used: 'A female embryo', she speculates, 'could be developed just to the point where an ovary emerges and then the ovary could be cultured so that engineers could get eggs from it. The full woman would never be allowed to develop. Just her ovary.'

This is a terrible tale indeed. Few feminists would disagree with Corea's contention that patriarchal control over reproduction has tended to increase over the past century. But not all would agree that the scenario that Corea invokes is a necessary outcome for women, even if it is, at present, for agricultural animals. The first of her speculations is already coming true for cattle: scientists at the Agricultural and Food Research Council's Institute in Cambridge have managed to extract immature eggs from ovaries obtained from cows after slaughter, and to bring them to maturity in the laboratory. They could then be fertilised in vitro. For agriculture, this method offers financial advantages – many offspring at less cost – while avoiding the 'complications' of flushing embryos out of live cows.

Corea feels that, in a woman-hating society, women would become reproductive machines, like breeding cattle are now. Once the eggs are obtained from 'high-quality' women, perhaps kept specially for the purpose, the resulting embryos might be transferred into the wombs of other women. Scientists, Corea suggests,

> ... could immediately transfer the embryo into a woman in the lower 80 to 90 per cent of the female population. (These would be the breeders, the women who had been called 'surrogate mothers' in the early stage of the reproduction revolution when pharmacrats were conscious of the need for good public relations). The transferred embryo might gestate in the breeder for the entire nine-month pregnancy ... (Or), the engineers could transfer the embryo into a breeder, allow it to gestate for a certain number of months, and then remove the fetus by cesarian section at whatever point at which their incubators could take over.[12]

The prospect of such intensive control over our reproduction, and the denial of our choices, seems a chilling one. Yet we need to remember that such control need not rely on science and technology at all. Of course it is science and its methods that have yielded the knowledge about reproduction that results in the new technologies. But we do have to remember that patriarchy is just as capable of exerting control over our reproduction without the aid of technological wizardry. Just as chilling a scenario as Corea's is provided by Margaret Atwood's novel *The Handmaid's Tale*.[13] But Atwood's scenario invokes no technology controlling women's reproduction – just massively increased state control.

It is not clear from some feminist critiques exactly why we should expect that the technology will inevitably lead to women being farmed. The procedures involved in egg harvesting are, at present, largely experimental and rather difficult to control. However good individual medics are at the relevant techniques, the processes of bringing eggs to maturity and then harvesting them is a time-consuming and expensive procedure. So, for the moment at least, cost is likely to inhibit any large-scale 'harvesting' of human eggs by surgery as a means of controlling women's reproduction.

There is undoubtedly an economic incentive to farm cattle intensively through the use of egg harvesting techniques: the cost of laboratory production of mature eggs is outweighed by the profit to be obtained when the offspring mature. But why should men want to farm women? The only plausible reason for 'farming' women, as Corea suggests, would be to obtain eggs, perhaps for the creation of (boy?) babies to be developed wholly in the laboratory. In such a society, women as we know them would be non-existent. But it is not obvious why we should accept that such a future is likely. In the first place, we would need to explain why men should *want* to get rid of women, or just keep a few for eggs: we do, after all, provide patriarchy with all kinds of labour – usually at little or no cost. Second, this kind of future assumes that women can have no influence whatsoever on the development of technology or of future societies. That is a particularly pessimistic view of women's ability to resist.

On the other hand, as Corea points out, the techniques involved are ones that are currently available: it would, then, not take much to organise a suitable system to implement them. Corea's scenario relies on the assumption that, as technological interventions become more sophisticated, more controlling, (male) scientists will inevitably want to exert greater and greater control over the processes of reproduction. It is certainly true that, in very broad terms, the history of medicine has coincided with a history of greater control. That history, moreover, has largely been a history of increasing male control over women's role in reproduction; Mary O'Brien has argued[14] that it was men's discovery of their own role in paternity that led to patriarchal oppression of women. Men, she suggested, are distanced, alienated from the reality of reproduction and so seek ways to compensate.

Gena Corea uses O'Brien's argument to suggest a continuity between men's initial alienation from their role and modern reproductive technology. Corea argues:

> Reproductive technologies can do more than give males a sense of (genetic) continuity over time. They are transforming the experience of motherhood and placing it under the control of men. Woman's claim to maternity is being loosened; man's claim to paternity strengthened. Moreover, these techniques are creating for women the same kind of discontinuous reproductive experience men now have.[15]

They are indeed transforming the experience of motherhood. But need they be seen as so overwhelmingly controlling? Corea's use of O'Brien's arguments focuses specifically on the first part of her argument – namely, that men have long been alienated from reproduction. This in turn, O'Brien argued, created specific conditions of reproductive consciousness and practice. If men are indeed alienated, then that consciousness is likely, for men, to include a desire to control women's reproduction to the point where their own alienation ceases.

One aspect of that control is the development of technologies. But this, O'Brien suggests, brought in its turn a second dramatic change in reproductive consciousness and practice, particularly in relation to contraception. As she puts it, 'The freedom for women to choose parenthood is a historical development as significant as the discovery of physiological paternity. Both create a transformation in human consciousness of human relations with the natural world which must, as it were, be re-negotiated.'[16]

This second point is one that Corea omits to consider. Yet O'Brien's analysis raises two important points. First, this second revolution in reproductive consciousness is one that allows *women* greater control and choice. That is, women need not necessarily be the kinds of passive victims that Corea seems to portray. And second, O'Brien suggests that the second 'transformation of human consciousness' requires, not passive capitulation to greater control, but renegotiation. For feminists, that could include active resistance.

This second revolution has not been unequivocally good for women, of course. Some forms of contraceptive technology pose threats to our health (such as the contraceptive pill, or the IUD), and it is by no means clear that the 'sexual liberation' that followed the advent of the Pill in the 1960s was particularly liberating for women. But that is not the central point. O'Brien's argument is not so much that new discoveries in reproduction *determine* changes in social relationships, but that the new discoveries create the possibilities for us to change those relationships, both with others and with the natural world. New contraceptive technologies have, for example, transformed our relationship with our bodies, in the sense that they allow a decisive break between sexual practice and procreation.

It is indeed a pessimistic vision that sees, as Gena Corea does, an *inevitable* intensification of the social relations of patriarchy in the new reproductive technologies. Perhaps O'Brien's account of the first 'revolution in reproductive consciousness' is right, and men's domination of women increased as a result of realising the male role in fertilisation. But to assume that patriarchal domination will automatically increase further is a big assumption, and it begs two important questions. In the first place, it begs the question of what we mean by patriarchy;[17] and second, it begs the question of women's response.

A World Without Women?

As long as existing social arrangements (or similar) are around it seems unlikely that patriarchy would actually benefit from eliminating women altogether; we do, after all, provide reproductive services for free, and often at great cost to ourselves. Yet existing social arrangements may not persist. Indeed, one of the problems with thinking about women's resistance is that, in a society based on male power over us, our resistance can too easily encounter reaction. It is fear of that reaction that has led some feminists to refer to the risk of 'femicide':[18] one way of dealing with stroppy women as a means of reproducing future generations may be to get rid of them altogether.

Feminists writing about the fear of femicide have pointed to the woman-hatred that characterises patriarchal societies all over the world. From murder of widows and female infanticide, to selective abortion of female fetuses, evidence of the way women are despised is abundant. The possibility of preselecting the sex of our children may, critics have pointed out, lead to a marked selection of boys. It is not, at present, possible to select sex prior to fertilisation, by sorting sperm, say, despite occasional claims to the contrary. Even in agriculture, where there are strong economic reasons for biasing fertilisations towards one sex, no reliable method has yet been found. What is currently possible, however, is selective abortion of fetuses of the 'undesired' sex – and, of course, it may soon become possible to select sex at an earlier stage, by sexing embryos in IVF.

Most feminist writing on the possibility of sex selection have pointed to the extent of woman-hatred throughout the world, and to the extent to which there is clear evidence of a preference for boys. They have emphasised, too, that a society in which women are relatively scarce is likely to be one in which women have even fewer rights and privileges than we have now.

An alternative view is that sex selection might bring benefits, however morally reprehensible it appears. Some of these are not specific to women, such as the possibility of reducing the incidence of sex-linked genetic diseases which affect only boys, or the (rather more dubious) suggestion that every child would – if preselected for sex – be a wanted child.[19] Some alleged benefits may lend themselves to other, rather less desirable, ends such as the suggestion that enabling parents to select the sex of their child would reduce the birth rate in certain countries – which would in turn reinforce the message that poorer countries are poor merely because they are overpopulated.[20]

Yet another putative benefit is that feminists themselves could use techniques of sex preselection as a reproductive strategy – to produce a succession of daughters, say.[21] Mary Anne Warren sees this as a possible corrective tactic to a widespread preference for males, pointing out that some feminist groups in both Britain and the US are studying possible methods of conceiving girls rather than boys. She sees this tactic, however, as only a minor part of a wider struggle, pointing out that

> The use of sex selection may never be more than a minor part of the struggle against patriarchy . . . (but) it is not a substitute for any of the substantive goals of feminism. To the extent that these goals are met, interest in selecting sex will decline. In the meantime, women will continue to resist male domination in innumerable ways, large and small; and these will sometimes include selecting the sex of their children.[22]

Yet should we accept such a technology on the grounds that we can resist some of its effects? It would not be a form of resistance that necessarily lends itself to furthering feminist demands, even if some of the individuals concerned are motivated by feminist ideals. As one critic pointed out,

> I cannot think of clearer examples of the instrumental use of children to further one's own agenda. And for every feminist who uses the technology to produce a nonstereotyped child, there will be ten others who produce children to fill precise sex roles.[23]

Ungrateful Women?

A central problem with thinking about how women might resist is separating out the kinds of resistance that might be useful *now* – in the kind of society we now have and to the kinds of technology we now have, or which are imminent –

with the kind of resistance that might become necessary if radically new developments (cloning, for example) become possible.

Underlying much feminist writing about fears for women's future is a vision of patriarchy – male domination – that is always the same. It changes historically only to the extent that it progressively gets worse. So, just because the technology for extracting embryos and transferring them exists now, we are led to believe that it will inevitably be used by men specifically to control women's lives. But the trouble with that view is that 'male domination' in our society is not so simple – even if they could, men would not necessarily want to control women in quite such a single-minded fashion because it is not in their interests to do so. Women currently provide cheap labour within a capitalist society; why should we suppose that men would want to lose that? Indeed, that is a central problem with the 'farming' scenario; it confounds the present with the future. We cannot assume that, say, cloning and ectogenesis *would* in practice be particularly desirable, even to a future patriarchy that wanted to control women.

It is equally unclear why a future society – even a highly inegalitarian one – should want to use reproductive technologies to create a specific class of creatures for, say, menial work. Why should we assume that a future society would want to spend large sums of money on such a project as cloning masses of people, say? For what purpose would such armies of identikit people be created? Tedious repetitive work is increasingly being taken over by machines because it is cheaper to do so; and if a future society wanted to use cloning to create specific classes to service the rulers or to rule themselves, then cloning would not necessarily be enough. However identical the genes, they do not ensure that different individuals react identically to different environments. Above all, identical genes do not guarantee docility: machines would surely be safer.

Equally, it is hard to see why even the most exploitative of societies should want to create hybrids. The science fiction image of half-human creatures is one in which they are kept by the ruling species (pure humans) to do the tedious tasks required by the society. But even if a relatively cheap technology existed to mass-produce such creatures, they would still cost more than machines to maintain. Besides, capitalism has little need to go to the expense of creating them: it has managed perfectly well with class, gender and race divisions for several centuries.

These possibilities terrify us: but we have also to remember that our terror is based on techniques that are being tried now. We cannot predict what techniques may become available in the future. Consider, for instance, the discussion of what may happen to women if the technology for preselecting the sex of a child were to become widely available. Feminist assessment of this future has always presupposed that our biological sex is a given, determined by our chromosomes at fertilisation. But imagine the kind of society we might have in the future if

> ... current developments in biomedical engineering, especially genetic engineering, make it quite likely that one day people will be able to spend part of their lives as men and part as women. Nature has already solved this problem, for, in certain species of fish, breeding males can change into breeding females, and vice versa. One day [techniques of manipulating embryos] may permit the mammalian reproductive system likewise to regress and redifferentiate.[24]

This rather bizarre suggestion is extremely unlikely, at least in the foreseeable future (and may never be possible). But it does remind us of the need for caution in extrapolating to the future from what we know of biological or technological possibilities now. Selecting sex becomes a problem for feminists because it is an either/or decision. In the (unlikely) event that human development could be tinkered with so that changing sex was easy, then the problems may be different.

Indeed, we can assess only those technologies that we have now, or might have imminently, because any technological development has to be considered within whatever social arrangements exist at the time of its invention. As those social arrangements change over time, so will the social relations in which a technology is used. And, in turn, the conditions in which *further* modifications and developments of that technology are pursued will change, too. Current Western society – patriarchal and capitalist – has its own way of reproducing: this relies on parents to pay the costs and on women within the family to do the work. Within these arrangements, substituting expensive (and sometimes faulty) technology for women's (cheaper) labour makes little sense.

Not only do we know nothing of future social organisation, we also know nothing of what technologies may become possible. There is no doubt that patriarchal control *could* increase as reproductive technologies develop. But they also may not, and we must beware of assuming a slippery slope into the future. Different technological developments – such as techniques enabling people to change sex even in reproductive terms – could lead to technological and social developments that we cannot foresee.

Politically, that slippery slope implies that our only recourse is to reject all reproductive technologies out of hand, in order to safeguard the future – a quest which, in practice, seems rather hopeless. One of the central problems politically with rejecting all reproductive technologies on the grounds of our fears of what men may do in the future is, we would argue, that it does not give us clear political direction *now*, to deal effectively with the technologies we have already. While techniques such as IVF and prenatal diagnosis clearly do present feminists with challenges, it is important for feminist strategy that we do not confound those, more immediate challenges, with hypothetical threats to women's reproductive role in some distant future.

We would argue that confounding the present – which undoubtedly raises questions for feminism in relation, say, to practices involved in IVF or in prenatal diagnosis – with a nebulous future serves us ill. Despite the misogyny in medical practices, we have no good reason to believe that we are on a slippery slope towards a society in which all women are denied the right to bear children; the driving forces – economic, political and ideological – are lacking. It is fear of that future that leads to total rejection: but it is not a helpful strategy for feminists, we suggest. What seems more important is to develop more specific strategies for dealing with specific technologies and how they affect the lives of different women: total rejection may not always serve the needs of all women equally.

Developing strategies has to take into account different forms of resistance, and differing needs. The increase in technological management of labour, for example, has certainly taken away much of women's dignity, and has contributed in some cases to greater problems for our children. But there are always some women for whom hospital, high-tech deliveries have saved their lives, for whom technology has been wonderful. Women, moreover, have not taken the technology lying down. As Ann Oakley has pointed out,[25] what perplexes many medics is just how *ungrateful* we are that all this technological wizardry is on offer: surely we should accept it without qualms? One problem facing anyone involved with health education campaigns, such as encouraging women to come forward for cervical smears, is that – for various reasons – women are *not* always 'grateful' nor passively accepting. New technologies may not be bad for all women: and women have always found ways to resist.

9. Official Attitudes to Reproductive Technologies in Britain and Elsewhere

One of the few things on which nearly every interested party seems to be agreed is that the law needs to catch up with developments in science and reproductive technology. Implicit in this is the idea that such things *should* be regulated, that they cannot just be left to scientists, doctors and the people they treat. As we saw in Chapter Two, according to the liberal idea of science as the progressive accumulation of value-neutral knowledge, scientists are supposed not to let their values colour their research. Therefore, the day-to-day practice of science should not be affected by ethical considerations, nor should scientists be required to set the overall ethical guidelines for their research or clinical practice; the content of such guidelines is not a scientific but a moral and political issue, in which scientists have no particular expertise. According to this popularly held view, it is up to philosophers and spiritual leaders to sort out the moral and ethical problems and for politicians, as legislators, to embody these in laws that effectively regulate the practice of scientists.

In practice, as we know, doctors and scientists do not have such a meek view of what they should be allowed to do. Indeed, the women's health movement has arisen largely as a result of the criticism that doctors frequently arrogate to themselves the right to decide who to treat and what treatment is suitable for them. This, as we have seen, has been a particular problem for women with regard to reproductive choices. The law often enshrines the right of doctors to decide; the most pertinent example of this is the requirement that two doctors certify that a woman's grounds for an abortion come under those allowed by the 1967 Abortion Act. Doctors have jealously guarded their right to decide, defending it simultaneously from the claims of both the law, when, for example, attempts have been made to impose a shorter time limit on abortions, and from the 'patients' themselves, resisting the feminist proposal for abortion on demand.

So why then have doctors and scientists been prominent among those pushing for legislation? Some would argue that this is just a public-relations exercise: that scientists would prefer a free hand but, in an attempt to dispel an image of themselves as dangerous and unprincipled, they make concessions to the opposition.

A related view is that scientists and doctors are worried about a reaction, that they expect to be attacked for their research on early embryos by the fundamentalist, anti-abortion lobby and other traditionalists. In such circumstances to have the fall-back of legal protection, to be able to say that they have not breached the law, would be useful. Coupled with this, particularly in the US, but increasingly so in this country, is the fear of malpractice suits, whereby patients have tried to sue their physicians for astronomical sums for having failed, for example, to alert a pregnant woman to a possible genetic defect in her fetus. To have clear legal guidelines would avoid some of such cases and certainly reduce the costs of fighting others.

But it is not only the medical profession that has been pressing for legislation. Pressure groups both for and against the new developments have formed to promote legislation in the direction they favour. Politicians, however, have been remarkably slow to legislate. Perhaps because of the strength of feeling such pressure groups display and the support that can be whipped up in their constituencies, politicians may feel that any action in either direction may succeed in losing them votes from one organised lobby or another. For example, President Reagan effectively ducked the issue, by failing to appoint a successor to the Commission on Bioethics he dissolved in March, 1985 – a move which has effectively stopped all publicly funded embryo research in the US, because by law it would have to be approved by such a body.[1] And in Britain, although the Warnock Committee reported in 1984, no legislation based on it was proposed by the government until 1987, just after they had won a General Election.[2]

The pressure groups divide along expected lines. Traditionalists have been pressing for legislation, largely in an attempt to ban anything that seems to threaten the status quo. In particular, because of their connection with the anti-abortion movement, they have focused on embryo experiments, which they see as raising a similar threat to the sanctity of life. They have criticised all forms of infertility treatment that use technology; they have questioned the propriety of the introduction of third parties, doctors, into the private matter of reproduction; they have disliked the involvement of donors; and they have displayed an immediate revulsion towards any form of surrogacy. In all cases, their dislike of a practice has meant that they have wished to ban it or at least regulate and curtail its availability. Tending to be allied with the more authoritarian wings of conservatism, particularly with respect to the family, tolerance of others who participate in practices they themselves find distasteful has never been the hallmark of this particular brand of right-wing thought.

Opposing them are the progressives, those who believe that on the whole good should be expected to come from the promotion of research and new forms of clinical treatment. They too are ultimately in favour of legislation to prevent abuses, but feel they can take their time. In practice, they have been most concerned to prevent hastily devised legislation being passed to outlaw research. They claim support from the medical profession, those campaigning for the handicapped, the birth control lobby and many feminist organisations.

Feminists in general, however, have been more ambivalent about legislation. Even those who reject current reproductive technologies, and fear that they are but the precursor of much more sinister future developments, have mixed feelings about the use of the legislative process as a way of stopping them. And those who support the pro-research view are even more dubious as to what is to be gained from legislation. This is for two reasons. First, most feminists, in Britain at least, have seen the law and law-making as largely dominated by men, who pass legislation that directly or indirectly bolsters their existing power: in other words, they see the state as not a neutral instrument but one reflecting the male-dominated power structure of society. They therefore doubt whether any good could come of regulations laid down by such a state. Similar ambivalences have been shown over sentencing for rape. On the one hand, feminists have criticised the attitude of male judges who pass lenient sentences for such a serious crime. On the other hand, it is not clear that more power to imprison for such judges and longer sentences for rapists is the answer.

The other reason why feminists have been more half-hearted than most about the idea of legislating on reproductive technologies has been a fundamental commitment to 'reproductive freedom'. This, as we have seen throughout this book, has in general led feminism to take a permissive stance with respect to reproductive choice, seeing individual women as the appropriate people to decide upon the use of their own bodies for reproductive purposes, rejecting the idea that any other party has a legitimate interest in such decisions. Thus the slogan, coined in defence of abortion:

> Not the church, not the state,
> Women must decide their fate

cannot easily be suspended when it comes to reproductive choices made by infertile women, even by those who have strong doubts about the benefits of the treatment such women are being offered. Feminists could, however, demand that the state help women to achieve that goal; legislation that guaranteed women the right to infertility treatment, whatever their marital status, sexuality or race, and an obligation on the NHS to provide such treatment, would be moving in that direction. But the sort of legislation generally under discussion, which bans or regulates certain reproductive choices, is difficult for feminists to support, whatever their own worries about the exploitative or discriminatory character of current practices or fears about where they might lead in the future.

This has been particularly true in Britain, where so much feminist attention has been focused on the defence of abortion and where anti-abortion forces have ensured that other issues, such as whether to allow experiments on embryos, are fought out on the same terrain. But even in Australia, where the women's movement is much more critical of new reproductive technologies, the most feminists have asked for in legislative terms is a moratorium on future developments while current practice is assessed.[3]

In the United States, feminism has tended to favour an enlargement of the concept of reproductive rights, though there often the issues are fought out in the courts rather than the legislature.[4] While formal freedom may be easier to gain and discrimination easier to challenge than in this country, the absence of a national health service means that access to treatment may in practice be much more unevenly spread. There the New Right has so far failed to restrict the legal availability of first and second trimester abortions, but has managed to prevent public funds being spent on providing such abortions. So while in Britain, women have to plead with their doctors for their 'reproductive rights', US courts up to now have considered the right to choose in such circumstances an automatic part of their 'right to privacy'.[5] Nevertheless, women in Britain may have less difficulty obtaining abortions than women in the US, who have had their right to reproductive choice curtailed by a lack of provision of services, particularly in rural areas, and by legislation which allows Medicaid funding for childbirth but not abortion.

Warnock and After

It was against a background of clamour for something to be done about reproductive technologies that the Warnock Committee of Inquiry into Human Fertilisation and Embryology was set up in July 1982 'to examine the social, ethical and legal implications of recent, and potential developments in the field of human assisted reproduction'. The committee consisted mainly of professionals potentially involved in 'the field', doctors, lawyers, social workers and administrators, but its chair, Mary Warnock, was an eminent philosopher. It included no representative of women's organisations nor any specific representatives of any religion, though there was at least one Jew and one Catholic on the committee as well as a professor of social and pastoral theology. In the course of its deliberations, the committee collected evidence from almost 700 organisations and individuals.

The Warnock Committee's report, published in 1984,[6] was not the first report in the world into the use of new reproductive technologies and the research behind them. Indeed, in Britain, both the Medical Research Council and the Royal College of Obstetricians and Gynaecologists had produced their own reports before the Warnock Report was published. But it has proved extremely influential world-wide, and a study carried out at Georgetown University in Washington of fifty such reports published throughout the world up to September 1986 found Warnock to have had a great influence on the major reports of all Western nations and Japan.[7] It is therefore worth looking in some detail at the issues it tackled, the background to them and the subsequent debate generated.

The Warnock Report's main proposal was to set up a

licensing body to give guidance on and regulate, through the ability to grant or withhold licences, research involving human embryos and various forms of new and not so new infertility treatments. Unlicensed practice would then become a criminal offence as well as certain other practices which the committee wished to rule out from the start, such as research on embryos more than fourteen days old or cloning. The legality of other practices would be left to the licensing authority's discretion; any that it decided against it could refuse to license.

The government was slow to act, and explicitly postponed legislation until after the 1987 election. In November 1987, the government announced its proposals for legislation but still only in the form of a White Paper,[8] rather than a specific Bill. The White Paper includes some, but not all, of the Warnock Committee's recommendations, but fails to take a clear position on the politically contentious issue of embryo research, suggesting instead a free vote for MPs between two alternatives: either to allow it up to fourteen days, as Warnock had recommended, or to ban it completely. Despite previous government assurances to the contrary, no legislation was proposed in its first two years of office. So if, as now looks likely, a Bill is introduced in 1989/90 more than seven years will have elapsed since Warnock was set up before any resulting legislation gets to parliament.[9]

While the government has been dragging its heels, others have got in on the act. There have been a number of private members' bills to ban embryo research and to outlaw surrogacy. Indeed, the latter issue provoked so much controversy that in July 1985 the government rapidly pushed through its own Surrogacy Arrangements Act, which banned commercial surrogacy agencies and advertising connected with any form of surrogacy. Since then there have been numerous attempts to make its provisions tighter, but none as yet has had any success.

In order to forestall further attempts to pre-empt Warnock and because it was clear that the setting up of the Statutory

Licensing Authority (SLA) would take a long time, the medical profession decided to set up its own system of control in the meantime. In 1985, the Medical Research Council and the Royal College of Obstetricians and Gynaecologists jointly sponsored the Voluntary Licensing Authority (VLA) for Human in Vitro Fertilisation and Embryology to license clinics and research centres according to its own guidelines, which were stated to be consistent with the Warnock recommendations and included the fourteen-day limit on embryo research. It approved twenty-four centres in its first year of operation and refused a licence to one.[10]

The VLA appeared at first to be as effective as any SLA would be, but it failed in 1987 to prevent one practitioner from putting women under increased risk of a multiple pregnancy. Ian Craft, of the private Humana Hospital in London, was transferring more than the maximum of three or four embryos recommended for IVF by the VLA. Craft claimed that those treating infertile couples should be able to exercise the same degree of clinical judgement as any other clinician, and that the VLA's attempts to control his practice were compromising the treatment of infertile couples for its own political ends. Other practitioners disagreed, claiming that Craft's techniques were placing other babies at risk as they competed for health service cots with premature quads born as a result of Craft's methods. His colleagues also worried about the politics of the situation: on tactical grounds alone, they thought he should be prepared to drop the most controversial techniques in order to prevent legislation being passed which would ban practices which they all supported.[11] When the VLA published its second report in 1987,[12] in which two new guidelines were added, against the insertion of more than three to four embryos and against the use of ova donated by relatives – all clinics, except Craft's, immediately agreed to toe the line. Craft, who had previously carried out both practices, temporarily lost his licence for refusing to agree to follow the new guidelines, but was subsequently granted a licence again when he agreed to comply. So the period of voluntary control, which is likely to come to an end with legislation, has demonstrated that professional self-regulation can lead to fairly effective control of specific 'excesses' which step outside guidelines that reflect current practice, but does not always work. Presumably, we can have much less confidence in the ability of even a statutory licensing authority to register concerns that go *against* existing practice or to engage in the much more difficult business of controlling the aims of research, about which most popular and feminist concern is expressed.

In terms of the issues discussed in this book, Warnock is relevant only to treatments for infertility and does not deal with prenatal diagnosis, though the use of AID and IVF with donated eggs or embryos to prevent the transmission of hereditary disease without the need for abortion is discussed, and the prevention or treatment of such diseases mentioned as one of the possible benefits of embryo research. Because no one had suggested banning amniocentesis or other forms of prenatal testing, the main legislative issue involved here is the availability of abortion, particularly of late abortions. Existing abortion law provided a 'necessary point of reference in discussions' of the Warnock Committee, so it would seem sensible to look at this issue first.[13]

Abortion Law and Prenatal Testing

Under the Offences Against the Person Act, all abortions had been made illegal in England and Wales in 1861, though in practice they were performed occasionally in public hospitals to save the mother's life. It is not, of course, possible to know how many illegal abortions were performed, but estimates in the 1930s varied from 50,000 to 250,000 per year.[14] These were of two types: expensive ones performed by qualified doctors and less expensive ones performed by unqualified, back-street abortionists. Although the latter were often highly experienced, the illegal circumstances in which they had to operate inevitably made abortion a dangerous procedure for all but the wealthiest of women. Over 500 women were reported as having died in 1933 as a result of illegal abortions, and the real number must have been much higher since there was known to be significant under-reporting of this illegal cause of death.[15]

From the 1930s, organised pressure groups started to campaign for a liberalisation of abortion laws. A brave decision by the eminent gynaecologist, Aleck Bourne, to perform an abortion on a fourteen-year-old girl who had been raped and then inform the police of his actions, led to a trial in 1938 at which he was acquitted on the grounds that it was impossible to distinguish a danger to life from a danger to health. Because the 1861 Act referred to unlawful abortions, there had to be some circumstances in which abortion was lawful, and the jury decided that this was such a case. This left the law in an uncertain state. It appeared to allow abortion for the sake of a woman's health, including mental health; but the case never went to appeal and so was never tested in higher courts. Nevertheless, other cases went the same way and gradually doctors became more willing to carry out such abortions.

By the 1960s there was increasing pressure for legislative reform. Tragically, but interestingly, from the point of view of this discussion, it was the issue of fetal handicap which seems to have precipitated public recognition of the need for reform. In the early 1960s, it became clear that a drug, thalidomide, which had been given to large numbers of pregnant women suffering from nausea, had caused severe deformities in the babies they subsequently bore. Hundreds of women, who had already been given the drug, then sought abortions and were horrified to find that abortion in such circumstances was illegal. It was the fate of these respectable women which raised the level of public debate. No longer did abortion appear to be inevitably associated with illegal and unhygienic practices. It became something that 'innocent' women could be asking of their doctors, for reasons large numbers of people could sympathise with. By July 1962, a national opinion poll found that 73 per cent of the population was in favour of abortion where the child might be born deformed.[16]

Nevertheless, it took a succession of failed attempts to get private members' Bills through parliament before David Steel's Abortion Act in 1967 was passed. No party had been prepared to support abortion reform, so it was left to private members to steer their own bills through the mire of parliamentary procedure, just as since then it has been private members' Bills which have tried to amend and restrict the Act. Nevertheless, opinions on abortion did roughly follow party lines: Labour and Liberal MPs, with the exception of Roman Catholics, being more likely to be in favour of reform together with a much smaller number of progressive Conservatives, while more right-wing Conservatives and the religious, both Catholics and fundamentalist Protestants, were opposed. This line-up, as we shall see, is a familiar one which has been repeated throughout subsequent debates on abortion and issues concerning reproduction.

The 1967 Abortion Act also set a pattern which subsequent proposals for legislation on reproductive issues have followed. It gave *doctors* the power and responsibility to decide whether the reasons of a woman wanting an abortion were acceptable grounds within the Act, even when they were effectively deciding about a woman's social circumstances. The Act also required that all abortions be notified to the Medical Officer of Health and set up a government-run *licensing and inspection system* for clinics outside the NHS wishing to perform abortions. The Department of Health, which was to grant such licences, was also to set the grounds on which licences could be revoked. It could change these grounds by Statutory Instrument, that is without recourse to parliament, as the prevailing climate on abortion changed. Indeed, it has occasionally done so, for example in 1975, restricting the type and number of clinics that could offer abortions after twenty weeks.

These aspects of the 1967 Abortion Act were seen by most abortion reformers as unnecessary restrictions, based on prejudice rather than the welfare of the women concerned. Nevertheless, they became part of the Act in an attempt to allay opponents' fears that abortion was a dangerous operation, whose legality could give rise to substantial 'abuses'. Bureaucratic hurdles and the implication that abortion was legal only in certain circumstances went some way to placating traditionalist opinion, though it had no effect on hard-line Catholic opposition. Interestingly, one of the principles supported by opponents, that abortion be considered legal if it was safer for a mother's health than continuing with the pregnancy, has in practice provided the grounds which have enabled liberal doctors to give women some measure of autonomy in their reproductive choices. For, except in very late pregnancy, abortion has a lower maternal mortality rate than childbirth, allowing those grounds to apply in practically any case. It was prejudice against abortion which convinced its opponents that it was an inevitably dangerous procedure that led to them allowing that relatively liberating clause to be passed.

What the 1967 Abortion Act did not do was ensure that all women qualifying under its grounds could actually get abortions, and the proportion of abortions performed in the NHS has been falling ever since; only 46 per cent of abortions on women resident in England and Wales in 1986 were performed within the NHS.[17] Most women needing abortions now have to go to expensive private clinics or to one of the non-profit-making clinics run by the abortion charities. These charitable clinics were started as a temporary expedient, while NHS facilities expanded, to satisfy the anticipated excess demand for abortions after 1967; since then, in practice, they have come to play an increasingly important role in providing abortions for those who cannot afford private medicine. It is not known how many women fail to negotiate all the hurdles of the Abortion Act and do not manage to get an abortion. The Lane Committee, set up in 1971 to investigate the workings of the Act, estimated that 30 per cent of those asking for National Health Service abortions did not get them and that about one third of these turned to the private sector. Many women go straight to the private sector, not wishing to face the humiliating process of pleading their case to an unsympathetic GP. An element of the unfairness of the system has always been regional disparities in the availability of abortion. In some parts of the country it remains nearly impossible to get an NHS abortion, because of the hostility of local gynaecologists, while in other parts it is relatively easy.[18]

There are two types of grounds allowed by the Act. One type refers to the needs of the woman and her family and allows abortion where the continuance of the pregnancy would involve a risk to the pregnant woman's life or to her physical or mental health or that of her family, greater than if the pregnancy were terminated. It is the inclusion of considerations of mental health and effects on the woman's family that leads the Act to be described as allowing abortion on both medical and social grounds. But, as can be seen, the terminology is purely medical and this coupled with the requirement that the grounds be certified by a registered medical practitioner gives doctors considerable power in their interpretation of the Act. The other ground on which abortion can be certified as necessary is where 'there is substantial risk that if the child were born it would suffer from such physical or mental abnormalities as to be seriously handicapped' and it is this clause which has allowed 'therapeutic abortions' for abnormal fetuses and has led to the development and use of prenatal screening for fetal disability.[19]

The Act was passed before the current wave of feminism was under way. But those who campaigned for it, such as the members of the Abortion Law Reform Association, supported what today we would call a feminist position on this issue. Since the Act's passage, feminists have been active in its defence, at the same time as being critical of its limitations.

Positive legislation has been proposed at various times to allow abortion on demand and to force the National Health Service to meet the demand for abortions. But such legislation has either failed to reach parliament or, once there, to jump the hurdles of parliamentary procedure, and so has never had a chance to be tested by a serious vote.

Instead, feminists have had to put their energies into the defence of this imperfect Act, in the face of persistent attempts to weaken its provisions. In the twenty years since its passage, at least ten serious attempts have been made in parliament to amend it: to impose a time limit on legal abortions, to restrict the grounds on which they are allowable, or to put further bureaucratic obstacles in the paths of women seeking abortions. All so far have failed, including the most recent attempt by Liberal MP David Alton, which had looked as though it might succeed in its aim of restricting the availability of late abortions.

Alton's Bill was presented to the House of Commons on 27 October 1987, the twentieth anniversary of the 1967 Act, consisting of a single clause, making all abortions illegal after eighteen weeks, except when the mother's life was in danger. Though Alton, as a Catholic, is against all abortions, his aim in putting forward such a simple bill was tactical. It was to prevent it, like many previous attempts to amend the Abortion Act, being 'talked out' by opponents proposing amendments and insisting that they get debated until the allotted parliamentary time is exhausted and the Bill automatically falls. Nevertheless, amendments were made, including an exemption from the eighteen week rule for women found to be carrying a fetus suffering from a severe disability. Thus the medical lobby, which was most incensed by the prospect of fetal disabilities being discovered by amniocentesis too late for legal abortion, was partially placated by this amendment.

The issue of whether or not to support such an amendment caused some disagreement among feminists. On the one hand, some argued that: 'We find it completely hypocritical that some doctors will carry out late abortions only when 'fetal abnormality' is diagnosed in the belief that some babies are worth less than others.'[20]

If the law decides it is too late to abort a normal fetus, then to allow abortion of abnormal fetuses is a form of eugenic discrimination against the disabled. This seems to be the position supported by the Women's Reproductive Rights Campaign: 'If the time limit is to be set at 24 weeks, we *cannot condone* the exemption of 'abnormal' fetuses from the time limit.'[21]

On the other hand, it would be extraordinary for feminists not to support an amendment that would allow at least some of the women seeking late abortions the right to choose.

Like all other attempts so far to amend the Abortion Act, David Alton's Bill to ban late abortions failed. This means that therapeutic abortions on the basis of prenatal diagnosis, like late abortions on the other grounds allowed under the Act, remain legal. It does look likely, however, that in the near future, some Bill to restrict women's access to abortions after twenty-four weeks, if not earlier, will be passed. The 1967 Act specified no time limit. Instead it made reference to the 1929 Infant Life Preservation Act which considered a fetus to be viable at twenty-eight weeks. Advances in the care of premature infants have led most doctors to interpret that limit as more like twenty-four weeks now, and, indeed, some attempts have been made to enforce that time limit. Since 1985, private clinics have not been licensed to carry out abortions except in emergencies over twenty-four weeks and the number carried out in NHS hospitals has been extremely low (twenty-five in 1986, only four in the second quarter of 1987).[22] The result of this intertwining of laws about two quite different things has been that the development of expensive technology which occasionally succeeds in keeping a very premature baby alive has been allowed indirectly to curtail women's rights, in quite other circumstances, to choose abortion.

A Select Committee of the House of Lords recognised the

absurdity of the way late abortions are currently prevented when it recommended dropping a proposed Bill to amend the Infant Life Protection Act so that a fetus be presumed viable from twenty-four weeks.[23] Recognising that the real intention behind the Bill was to restrict the availability of late abortion, it concluded that tampering with the Infant Life Protection Act was an inappropriate way to do so. It therefore set about making its own recommendations on late abortions, and proposed that reference to the Infant Life Protection Act be removed from the Abortion Act, thus abolishing any overall time limit, but that the grounds under which abortion after twenty-four weeks be allowed should be considerably narrower than those for earlier abortions. The storm of outrage from conservative and 'pro-life' peers provoked by this honest attempt to interpret the true intentions of the 1967 Abortion Act shows how far we have come from the days of liberal paternalism in which it was passed. The members of the committee should be congratulated on the stand they took in these illiberal times, even though it too falls far short of letting women make their own choices as to when and in what circumstances late abortions are permissible. Again, as in all such debates, late abortions on grounds of fetal abnormality, rather than the needs of the woman, are those which provoke least hostility and which are often used to argue against the imposition of any blanket prohibition on late abortions.

Prenatal testing with a view to 'therapeutic' abortion also raises the issue of whether treatment can be withdrawn from severely disabled new-born babies. In the United States, there is no legal right to withhold treatment at the request of parents. But in Britain a doctor, Leonard Arthur, prosecuted in 1981 for allowing a severely handicapped baby to die, as the parents had asked, was acquitted because a large number of eminent doctors gave evidence to the effect that his actions were in accordance with general medical practice.[24] But in neither country is the provision of such treatment guaranteed by the state, and British parents have failed in the courts to get life-saving heart operations provided by the cash-starved NHS in time to save their babies' lives.[25]

Finally, the contentious issue of sex-selective abortion is definitely not legal under the British Abortion Act; though presumably it is, at least at an early stage of pregnancy, in the US. Following an investigation, by Channel Four's 'Eastern Eye' in June 1985, of private clinics alleged to be doing abortions on grounds of fetal sex, the DHSS circulated all licensed clinics pointing out that such grounds do not qualify under the 1967 Act. Despite this, the *Sunday Times* claimed that such abortions were still being done on some Asian women by a few private clinics in May 1986.[26] But sex selection may soon become possible without needing to fall foul of abortion law. In December 1986, a baby born after IVF in Italy was said to be the first test-tube baby in the world whose sex had been chosen. And in August 1987, Patrick Steptoe claimed that he would shortly make the screening of embryos for sex generally available to couples seeking IVF at his clinic.[27]

Donation of Gametes and Embryos

The other practice that had been widely debated long before Warnock was the donation of sperm for artificial insemination. This had been a technological possibility for a very long time, but became a relatively common 'treatment' for male infertility only after the Second World War. The first known use of artificial insemination was in Scotland in 1790, when a linen draper's sperm was successfully used to inseminate his own wife. This was in fact fifty years before scientists understood that for fertilisation to occur a sperm must enter a woman's egg, showing that then, as now, the development of a technique can pre-date the scientific understanding of the biology that makes it work. Despite this success, it was nearly 100 years before the first recorded use in 1884 of *donor* sperm to impregnate the wife of an infertile man in Philadelphia. The few recorded cases of the use of artificial insemination by donor

(AID) in the following fifty years are notable more for the prurient curiosity and moral censure they occasioned than as evidence that the practice was spreading.[28]

During the 1930s, some infertile couples were helped by a few doctors willing to practise AID in a number of Northern European countries, the United States and Canada. But there is no way of knowing how extensive its use was, as AID was practised extremely secretively in the face of considerable moral, theological and legal opposition. The children of such couples were formally illegitimate, though this can be assumed to have been hidden in most cases by the mother's husband being entered as the father on the child's birth certificate. Although doing so would have been illegal, there was no way it could have been found out, except when disputes subsequently arose. Where they did arise, however, AID was declared to be equivalent to adultery and thus grounds for divorce, for, according to a typical 1921 judgement: 'the possibility of introducing into the family of the husband a false strain of blood' was the defining characteristic of adultery not 'the moral turpitude of the act of sexual intercourse'.[29] This continued to be the legal position in most countries until quite recently; AID, even with a husband's consent, was adultery and any child so conceived was illegitimate.

In Britain, a paper published in the *British Medical Journal* in 1945, reporting on a number of cases where AID had been used, led to a storm of outrage. Its supporters saw it as a scientific solution to male infertility. But the popular press, appealing to an easily aroused distrust of scientists in the immediate aftermath of the first atomic bombs, warned of the eugenic possibilities of AID. The *Sunday Despatch* feared that 'a super-race of test-tube babies will become the guardians of atom-bomb secret'. Then, as now, fears about the dangers of science combined with a distaste of anything that might disturb the status quo, particularly where the family was concerned, to provide fertile ground for prejudice and intolerance.[30]

In 1948, a commission set up by the Archbishop of Canterbury recommended that AID be made a criminal offence. In 1951, Pope Pius XII condemned all artificial insemination on the two grounds that it necessarily involves the sin of masturbation for the donor, and that it severs the connection between sex and reproduction for the recipient. Further, the use of *donor* sperm is yet more reprehensible because it intervenes in the holy sacrament of marriage.[31] This remains official Catholic teaching, confirmed in a Vatican doctrinal statement in 1987. However, the more pragmatic Church of England, while reaffirming in 1960 its view that AID was undesirable and immoral, no longer advocated making it a criminal offence.

In 1960, a government enquiry, the Feversham Committee on Human Artificial Insemination, concluded that AID was an extremely unwholesome practice, but that it should not be made illegal for fear of driving it underground out of medical control.[32] They wanted the distasteful practice kept discreet, so that it should not spread. This report seems to have been a last ditch attempt by traditionalists to defend the family, already thought to be under threat from rising illegitimacy and divorce rates. AID was seen as a further attack on the institution of marriage and the relations of parents and children within it. Recognising that the practice could not be stopped, AID children had to be sacrificed to the defence of the status quo and should continue, like others whose biological parents did not marry, to be labelled illegitimate. 'Succession through blood descent is an important element of family life and as such it is the basis of our society. On it depend the peerage and other titles of honour, and the Monarchy itself', proclaimed the report of the committee whose chair was the current holder of the earldom of Feversham. And lest we suspect any class interest being involved, we were assured that this was a matter of vital importance, tantamount to the defence of the nation, which must concern us all: 'knowledge that there is uncertainty about the fatherhood of some is a potential threat to the security of all.'[33]

Although such reactions seem comical today, it is worth thinking why artificial insemination appeared to be such a threat. The Feversham Committee was, of course, right to say that family life lay at the basis of society. Capitalist societies, and some others, cope with the dependence and needs of children by parcelling them up into families, making their care a private matter to be allocated to particular individuals, usually their parents, rather than the responsibility of society of a whole. The obligation to provide for dependants is supposed to keep male, and increasingly female, bread-winners in line at the work-place, as well as providing an incentive for the accumulation of wealth to pass on to heirs. Illegitimate children, not being part of families, may force the state to provide some support, at least financially, and seemed, therefore, to threaten that system of family responsibility.

The Feversham Committee thought that this specific arrangement of capitalism was a biologically given one, based on an assumption that people are naturally willing to care for and pass on property only to children to whom they were genetically related. They were not unusual in this. Conservative thought has always tended to assume that the social arrangements that it favours preserving are based on nature (or god), rather than being the social expedients of a particular time and place. If current family arrangements were based on nature, rather than society, they could indeed be threatened if the natural processes which created families, and ensured that children were biologically related to their parents, were interfered with. The Feversham Committee viewed legitimacy in this light; rather than recognising it as pure social construct, they saw it as the legal recognition of a biological relationship. A relationship with no biological basis, like that between father and AID child, could not therefore be legitimated. In practice, this meant that the committee took the view that failing to make a relatively small number of infertile couples into proper families was less of a problem than allowing the identification of current social arrangements with nature to be broken down. Perhaps at the back of their mind too was the even more horrifying thought that if couples could use AID to acquire children not biologically theirs, perhaps single women could bring children into households that made no pretence even of being proper families.

Indeed, more recent pronouncements have not been that different in their desire to preserve 'normal' family arrangements. The difference has been that the identification with biological parenthood has become less significant. Over the past twenty to thirty years, at the same time as a large increase in the number of stepfathers, there has been a gradual acceptance of the practice of AID, and thus a recognition that men in both situations are taking responsibility for children they have not biologically fathered. The Minister for Health decided in 1968 that AID and AIH should be made available within the NHS on medical grounds. However, despite this approval in principle, a survey by the Royal College of Obstetricians and Gynaecologists in 1977 found the funding of AID very patchy across the country.

By this time, the AID child, being wanted by both its parents, was seen as something quite different from the traditional illegitimate child who could not be assigned to a family. The former, therefore, did not pose the threat to family life that the latter had. Indeed, as more babies are born to unmarried, cohabiting couples, marriage and legitimacy is no longer so much the issue. The Law Commission, in its Working Paper on Illegitimacy, published in 1979,[34] sought to abolish the status by proposing that unmarried fathers be given the same parental rights and responsibilities as unmarried mothers, thus ensuring that all children be parcelled up into some family, however much of a fiction that family may be and whatever threat to the autonomy of women that may represent. But it specifically excluded AID children from this suggestion, to ensure that their position within the family was as much like that of a traditionally conceived child as possible. In other words, the Law Commission's concern, like that of the Feversham Committee, was to preserve family life. But in a spirit of realism, it recognised that the traditional unit of married biological parents and their offspring no longer have sufficient numerical dominance to consign all other forms to illegitimacy. The solution was to allocate all children to the best available approximation to that ideal. In finding this approximation for AID children, the traditional concern with a biological connection took second place to the equally traditional concern that parents be married, and legitimacy thus became shorn of any connection with biology, and effectively recognised for the social arrangement that it is.

Although AID is not a new technology, it was discussed at some length by the Warnock Report and used as the basis for its consideration of other forms of donation. It agreed with the Law Commission's view that AID children should be seen as the legitimate children of the mother and her husband, who should be allowed to register as the child's father, and that the donor should have 'no parental rights or duties in relation to the child'.[35] The child would be legitimate provided the husband had consented to the insemination, and a husband would be presumed to have consented unless he could prove otherwise, just as a husband is presumed to be the father of his wife's children unless he can prove otherwise. However, as good practice, they recommended that the consent of both partners be sought. The government's proposal for legislation based on Warnock also takes the view that a child, born as a result of any form of donation – of sperm, egg or embryo – to a married woman should be seen as the child of the marriage. They would thus legitimate the child for all laws governing the inheritance of property, but not, the Earl of Feversham will be pleased to note, for the succession to titles. This has in fact been the case for AID, in England and Wales, since the passage of the Family Law Reform Act in 1987, which took up some but not all of the Law Commission's 1979 Working Paper's suggestions.

Throughout the section on artificial insemination, the Warnock Report talks about the treatment of couples, and the consent of the man is seen as important to legitimate the child. This means that artificial insemination can create a new form of extra-family child, despite the general move to give unmarried fathers more connection with their children. Children born to a woman by artificial insemination, where no man has given his consent to the procedure, have no claim on any man. Warnock spends some time considering the position of children born from the frozen sperm of the mother's deceased husband, but presumably a much more usual case is that of a single woman choosing to have a child without a man's involvement. Indeed, if the proposals of the Law Commission's working party were ever accepted in full, and unmarried fathers were to be given all the same rights as mothers, which looks unlikely, then women would *have* to turn to AID if they wanted to have children without a man having an equal legal claim on them.

Another proposal of Warnock may make artificial insemination for women wishing to have children on their own more difficult to carry out legally, as the report recommends that AID be available only at licensed clinics and, by implication, that infertility services at such clinics should be provided preferentially to those in stable heterosexual relationships, though not necessarily married couples. But many women today arrange their own insemination. The Government proposals for legislation based on the Warnock Report would make this practice a criminal offence. This would be a serious incursion on women's reproductive freedom. It is also presumably quite unenforceable as far as private arrangements are concerned; who but the donor and recipient can be sure that insemination happened artificially and thus illegally, rather than naturally and perfectly legally? Even if mother and donor were subsequently in dispute, there appears little that either party could gain from revealing the truth.

On the other hand, the practical consequences are real. The services most likely to be curtailed are those offered by organisations such as the British Pregnancy Advisory Service, which currently arranges AID for women without making any moral judgements as to their suitability, and thus is one of the few clinics that will help lesbians and other less 'respectable' women who do not wish, or do not have the contacts, to arrange their own insemination. Whether such clinics will meet with the approval of the Statutory Licensing Authority remains to be seen. If they do not, the prospects for women who wish to have children with no direct contact with the father are poor, and even if licences are initially granted, the possibility that they might at some future date be revoked will always be an unwelcome restriction.

The Warnock Report does not see AIH (artificial insemination by 'husband', in practice meaning partner) as sharing any of the problems of AID, except its unnaturalness. And, despite wishing to invoke the criminal law if the latter is performed outside its licensed clinics, the report sees no reason for controlling the former at all. The distinction between AIH and AID is one that is significant only within the context of a couple, married or not. For a woman all artificial insemination is AID. Indeed, for a woman artificial insemination is biologically no different from the natural process. The focus of discussion and the deliberate separation of AIH, as a relatively unproblematic procedure, from AID, a procedure fraught with difficulty, reflects men's concerns about it. Women may have all sorts of things to gain from artificial insemination, including the choice to have children on their own and the possibility of avoiding passing on genetic defects without repeated abortions.

It is only recently that the issue of egg donation has come up as a possibility too. It is a much more difficult procedure than sperm donation and cannot be carried out without medical involvement. The Warnock Report accepts egg donation as following logically from its acceptance of AID and suggests the same licensing arrangements and procedures of anonymity. It also recommends that the legal mother be the recipient, not the donor, and that donors should have no subsequent rights or responsibilities to the child, in line with its view on the role of sperm donors. Although the conduct of the debate and the formal solutions proposed may be the same in the two cases, the questions raised will in practice inevitably be very different, not only because of the relative difficulties of the procedures involved, but also because paternity and maternity do not have the same status in our society or raise the same issues.

The Government's White Paper talks about the donation of sperm and eggs (and even embryos) interchangeably as if there were no difference between the two – though Warnock did not, recognising that in practice there is a great deal of difference. The dangers and difficulties of egg donation mean that although women may be willing to undergo a donation operation to help a friend or a sister, it is much less likely that they will be persuaded to become anonymous egg donors or that egg banks will be set up to be supplied by Nobel prizewinning women. Anonymous donation may be seen as acceptable for women undergoing other operations, but even so the process of egg donation may still seriously inconvenience them. Recipients of eggs will have much less choice than recipients of sperm about their donors and may have to persuade friends or relatives to become donors. This means that inevitably questions are begged about the pressures that might be put on women to donate eggs, either by the medical profession, while undergoing other treatment, or by other members of their family.

Warnock, with a view to 'minimising the invasion of a third party into the family',[36] recommended that all donors be anonymous, except where specific private arrangements were made, such as those between sisters or brothers. Without specifically approving of it, Warnock thereby recognised that in order to satisfy a desire to maintain a biological connection, it may be worth the risk of complicating family arrangements. But in general, anonymity was seen as the way to pretend that everything was normal. So, consistent with its general line, the Warnock Committee showed its concern with ensuring that children are born into families, and, adapting the law where necessary, gave the maintenance of biological links relatively little significance. The planned legislation, however, nowhere insists on anonymity, though it does presume it in making the proposal that a register of donors be kept, in order that they can be traced if, for example, a child is found to be the carrier of a hereditary disease. It rejects the suggestion, which now operates in Sweden, that children born as a result of AID should at the age of eighteen be able to find out the identity of the donor, though says that the child should have a right to know that he or she was born as a result of donation and certain 'non-identifying' information about the donor. In Sweden a law was passed in 1985 giving children the right to know the donor's name. Although this has not led to a long-term decline in the number of donors, it has led to a fall in the number of people seeking AID, suggesting that the need to draw inviolable bounds around the family may be a strong enough factor to discourage some women, or their husbands, from seeking help with infertility – or at least to seek help somewhere where Swedish law does not apply.[37]

The proposal for legislation treats all forms of donation, of sperm, eggs or embryos, in the same way. It also has a great deal to say about the storage of gametes and embryos, where inevitably there are a few differences, because embryos are created by a couple whereas gametes come from an individual. Currently only sperm and embryos can be stored, because eggs are damaged by freezing, but this problem is likely to be overcome in the next few years. Again, one of the main concerns of both Warnock and the subsequent proposal for legislation was about the rights of succession of any child born after the storage of gametes or sperm. The scenarios involving posthumous inheritance and so on take on a greater significance when storage is allowed, because the time lapse allows more and more anomalous situations to be created. This issue became extremely topical in Australia in 1983 when a wealthy childless Californian couple were killed in a plane crash leaving two embryos in a Melbourne freezer. The fate of the 'Rios twins' led to a spate of controversy about what should be done with such embryonic orphans, a controversy certainly fueled in part by interest in the massive fortune that would have been theirs if only they had been born. Public interest in this case led to the State of Victoria passing, in 1984, the first law in the world dealing with new reproductive technologies, the relevant clauses of which allowed freezing (cryopreservation) but discouraged long-term storage and required parents to decide in advance what to do in case of their death.[38]

Both Warnock and the proposed legislation wish to regulate the storage of gametes and embryos by setting up licensed 'storage authorities', specifying time-limits for storage and making unlicensed storage a criminal offence. Both see donors as having the right to specify the conditions of use of any stored gametes and, with the joint agreement of both donors, embryos. But there is a slightly different edge to their approaches, which can be seen in the insistence of the proposed legislation that the storage authority can exercise no control without the explicit instructions of the donors, whereas Warnock envisaged a number of situations in which the storage authority might become the effective guardian of the stored material. The government's proposals effectively give people individual or joint property rights in their own gametes or embryos, in contrast to Warnock's view that it was important that 'legislation be enacted to ensure that there is no right of ownership in a human embryo'.[39] This means that, whereas Warnock is prepared for non-familial embryos to have a storage authority as guardian, the government, perhaps reflecting a more right-wing traditionalist consensus, would rather have a neater solution with embryos preserved only if they have 'parents' willing to take responsibility for them.

However, none of the recent debates over egg and embryo donation have been anything like as intense as the earlier ones over AID. Because biological fatherhood is nothing but a genetic connection and social fatherhood can be such a tenuous connection, men, it seems, have been much more worried than women about becoming a parent to a child to whom they are not genetically related. A woman who uses a donated egg or embryo carries that child and will, under current social arrangements, still be that child's primary parent. She may indeed have less to worry about. The debates about AID seem to have reflected the traditional insecurity of men about the paternity of their children and their concern that their property be passed on to their own children. These have not been the traditional concerns of women who, after all, have had little property to pass on and no doubt about who their children were; nor on the whole have they been in a sufficient position of power to set the terms of such debates.

Today the concerns seem to have shifted. It is not so much the rights of inheritance as parental responsibility that concerns the lawmakers. Despite earlier attempts to claim biological inevitability for current social arrangements, there is now a general recognition that a biological connection is largely irrelevant to fulfilling a parental role. Modern debates and policy proposals reflect much more the concern that children be allocated to families that take responsibility for them, than the concern that children inherit from their own fathers. This marks a shift of emphasis from the conditions of reproduction of society's wealth-holders alone to those of the population as a whole. Such a shift may reflect the dwindling importance of who owns productive capital as it increasingly takes the form of large corporations run by managers rather than family businesses or landed estates, as well as an increased involvement of the state and social policy in the reproduction of the workforce.

Surrogacy

Similar concerns with the family have been apparent in moves to ban surrogacy, but here the passions aroused have been much stronger. These affected the Warnock Report too, which in its assessment of most other issues, followed a strictly rationalist approach. The Committee was 'mindful of the truth that matters of ultimate value are not susceptible of proof', but nevertheless they claimed to have formed their 'views on argument rather than sentiment'.[40] But when they came to surrogacy, their proposals seem to be based more on feeling than reason. Although, as on other matters, they give a reasoned summary of the arguments for and against, their proposals for legislation are all based, without evaluation, on the assumption that everything should be done to discourage surrogacy. Thus, for example, while recognising the grave dangers of exploitation of women inherent in commercial surrogacy, the majority rejected the proposal, supported by only two members of the Committee, of allowing the SLA to license non-profit making agencies to make non-exploitative surrogacy arrangements. And this proposal was rejected not on the plausible and relevant grounds that it might not succeed in avoiding exploitation, but because it 'would in itself encourage the growth of surrogacy'.[41]

Instead, they proposed banning all surrogacy agencies, profit-making or not, and further wanted to make any action that assists in bringing about surrogate pregnancy illegal. Although they did not see it as practicable to ban private surrogacy arrangements, they did wish to see the law explicitly ensuring that surrogacy contracts would not be enforceable. This is the case in existing law anyway in England and Wales, where the Children's Act of 1975 made it impossible for a person to transfer parental rights and duties to another person, rather than handing over the child to a recognised adoption agency. In other words, the surrogate mother does not anyway have the power to allow the commissioning parents to adopt her child, and certainly no one could enforce through the courts an agreement to hand over a baby.

The government's proposals also have as their main principle 'that legislation should not give any encouragement to the practice of surrogacy',[42] but they do not include any new legislation to ban it and do not propose making participation in non-commercial surrogacy agencies or arrangements a criminal offence. Thus the proposed legislation makes a distinction which most of Warnock rather surprisingly did not, between commercial and non-commercial surrogacy, and does not propose to criminalise the latter.

It does not need to act on commercial surrogacy because that has already been banned by a piece of legislation, the Surrogacy Arrangements Act, passed in July 1985, in reaction to public concern following a much publicised commercial surrogacy arrangement. Kim Cotton, acting as surrogate for an American couple arranged by the US-owned commercial 'Surrogate Parenting Agency', gave birth to a daughter in January 1985, amid huge publicity, much of which, it was suspected, Mrs Cotton had herself organised. Although custody of the child was not disputed, 'Baby Cotton' became the subject of a place of safety order by Barnet council and was subsequently made a ward of court, as a result of legal action brought by the commissioning parents. The High Court eventually ordered that the child be handed over by the council to the commissioning parents, at which point they flew her out of the country and out of the jurisdiction of British courts.

Despite numerous failed attempts by right-wing MPs to criminalise all surrogacy arrangements, and even to deny surrogate mothers the use of NHS facilities for the birth of their children, the current position is that privately arranged non-commercial surrogacy is legal but unreliable. Surrogacy contracts are unenforceable and adoption cannot be guaranteed, although commissioning parents can apply to the courts to adopt the child and, where there has been no dispute, have in practice been allowed to do so wherever they have been seen as providing a good home for the child. The issue of payment, however, could potentially lead to problems with this. The 1975 Children's Act does not allow adoption where any payment has been made for a child, although expenses can be paid. But, in 1986, a child was successfully adopted after a surrogate mother had been paid £5,000 'expenses' which allowed for emotional and physical factors as well as her loss of earnings. In another case in the same year, a surrogate mother who changed her mind was allowed to keep the twins she had borne and no question of repaying any fees came up in the court.[43]

A surrogacy arrangement can involve various combinations of genetic material, with either the egg or, more likely the sperm, coming from the commissioning couple; 'full' or 'true' surrogacy is when an embryo fertilised in vitro from sperm and egg provided by the commissioning couple is transferred to the surrogate mother. (The possibility that a single woman or man might commission a woman to bear a child for them is not even considered in the Warnock Report nor in any other official discussion of surrogacy, despite this being, in one form or another, the only method by which a single man could 'make' a child.) In all cases, the Warnock Report insisted that the surrogate mother, having carried the child, should always be taken to be the legal mother. This is biologically consistent with its position on donation, where donors have no parental rights or duties, though, of course, the different social relations of a surrogacy arrangement might suggest reversing the logic, putting the surrogate mother in the position of a donor or 'womb-leaser' as she has sometimes been called. However, going through with a surrogate pregnancy is quite different from donating sperm or eggs, and Warnock, quite sensibly, therefore recommends that changes in adoption law are a more appropriate way to regularise the situation of children born to surrogate mothers to whom they are not genetically related and subsequently brought up by their genetic parents.[44]

But despite considering this situation, the Warnock Report points out that its own proposals, which would make medical involvement in surrogacy illegal, would rule out any form which involves egg or embryo donation. If this were the case, only the current form of surrogacy could be practised, in which the man's sperm is the sole genetic contribution from the commissioning parents. Further, if the Warnock Report's other proposal, to make AID illegal except under the auspices of a licensed centre, were also to be accepted, such a surrogate pregnancy could be legally achieved only through intercourse, and surrogacy would be taken right out of the realm of technology. However, because such stringent legislation on surrogacy has not been proposed by the government, cases of these other 'fuller' forms of surrogacy may yet appear.

Thus Warnock adopted a completely different approach to surrogacy, compared with the way it considered other ways of alleviating infertility. In all other cases, its approach was to license and legalise under certain controls. For surrogacy, they moved back to the approach of the Feversham Committee and decided to do everything short of a total ban, which was thought counter-productive, to discourage the practice. Its distaste may be seen in the very language adopted. Whereas other practices are discussed as a solution for a couple's problem of infertility, the chapter on surrogacy talks mainly as though it was just the woman who might benefit, with the commissioning father getting a separate paragraph about his position. Although in general feminists might agree that these issues should be addressed more in terms of the individuals involved rather than the couple, it is strange that it is only in this one case that the Warnock Report does so. AID, for example, is seen as a solution for a couple, even though in this case the medical problem is presumably all the man's.

Other European countries have taken a similar attitude to surrogacy, often influenced by Warnock. In France, for example, surrogacy has been roundly condemned by the ethics committee set up by President Mitterrand to look at issues surrounding reproductive technology. Indeed it is thought that any intermediary could be found guilty of aiding the abandonment of a child, which is a criminal offence in France. And in West Germany, the Minister of Justice condemned surrogacy as 'the purest form of trafficking in human beings' and said the courts would categorically deny adoption papers to couples 'so pathological as to want to adopt a baby in this manner'.[45] Throughout the world, public opinion polls have found less than one third of their samples to have favourable attitudes to surrogacy, and all seven of the major governmental reports oppose it.[46]

In the US, on the other hand, commercial surrogacy agencies have been operating for some time; some of these operate internationally and have tried to set up offices in Europe. Several cases have come before the courts in the US, the most celebrated being that of 'Baby M'. Her mother, Mary Beth Whitehead, lost a legal battle over custody with the commissioning parents when she tried to keep the baby she had borne as a result of a surrogacy arrangement. This may be the first case in the world of a court's enforcing a surrogacy contract against the surrogate mother.[47] In its wake, some states have made surrogacy illegal, others have made surrogacy arrangements easier by simplified adoption procedures, while in a few states bills have been introduced to make surrogacy contracts enforceable.[48] In general, the climate in the US is less hostile to surrogacy than in Europe, more in favour of letting people do what they want if they can pay for it.

It is interesting to consider why this attitude is not more general, why surrogacy has provoked such a hostile reaction far beyond that shown to any other way of overcoming infertility. Perhaps one reason is that unlike other remedies, which can be hidden from view, surrogacy, like conventional adoption, must be a public event, even involving the courts if the legal position is to be straightened out. In this situation a normal family cannot really be the outcome, because the normal family should be a private product.

This lack of privacy happens with any adoption, but there are other factors in surrogacy too. With adoption, the best is being thought to be done for a child who has inadvertently fallen out of the family net. But in a surrogacy arrangement, a child has been voluntarily, and by implication wantonly, produced in these unfortunate circumstances. Further, a mother has willingly arranged to give up her child rather than being forced to by tragic circumstances. It is this which is perhaps particularly threatening. Underlying familial ideology is the picture of indissoluble bonds, those of marriage binding husband to wife, and, especially when marriage is no longer seen as so permanent, those of nature binding mother to child. Even if society has moved far enough to recognise that the bonds between husband and wife are no longer god-given, and those between father and child are more socially than biologically determined, it seems that the naturalness of the bond between mother and child is still taken for granted and anything which throws it into question is therefore to be rejected. The parallels with Feversham's rejection of AID are again apt. That committee saw AID as an abomination because it showed that men were willing to bring up children of whom they were not the natural fathers. Warnock rejects surrogacy because it shows that women are willing to part with their natural children. Although in both cases, it was the shift from a natural to a social relation that was disturbing, it is interesting that in the case of surrogacy the emphasis is on the unnaturalness of the woman who chooses *not to* bring up her child, while in the case of AID it is the man who chooses to raise another man's child who is seen as unnatural.

But although such a rejection of surrogacy is widespread, it is not unanimous. A minority position on the Warnock Committee saw surrogacy as a possibly beneficial solution for a few couples. Its two supporters suggested that surrogacy should be allowed under the control of the SLA, which would be able to license non-profit-making surrogacy agencies. They saw such agencies as similar to adoption agencies, with appropriate childcaring skills, and suggested that this was a role existing adoption agencies might be prepared to take on. They were also insistent that the arrangements must be non-profit-making, not so much because they were worried about commercial exploitation, either of the commissioning couple or of the surrogate mother, but because they saw the issues being the same as those surrounding adoption, where the law explicitly forbids any commercial transactions.[49]

The views of this minority are much more reasoned and in line with the tone of the rest of the Warnock Report than the majority position. For example, the minority statement talks of couples rather than just women as the beneficiaries from surrogacy, as the rest of the report does when considering other ways of alleviating infertility. But they do share with the majority a common feature of all pronouncements on surrogacy: a total rejection of the idea of it as a commercial arrangement. Why does the introduction of financial considerations invoke so much abhorrence in this case? One might think that it is a distaste for the idea of people making money out of others' misfortunes, but that is clearly not the case, as commercial arrangements are not disapproved of for other solutions to infertility. Warnock evinces concern for the possibility of exploitation of the surrogate mother:

> That people should treat others as a means to their own ends, however desirable the consequences, must always be liable to moral objection. Such treatment of one person by another becomes positively exploitative when financial interests are involved.[50]

But this statement is couched in such universal terms, that it makes one wonder on what basis its authors think our society normally runs.

It is clearly not money itself that is the problem, but that women are being paid for doing something that is normally part of the personal not the financial side of life. It is, as it is with prostitution, the mixing of money with what should, according to the norms of society, be done for other reasons, that leads to the distaste and the very real possibility of exploitation. Both surrogacy and prostitution constitute an overstepping of the boundaries between public and private, the introduction of the public way of getting people to do things by paying them money, into an activity which is supposed to remain within the private sphere. And even non-commercial surrogacy has some of that taint of overstepping boundaries; having children is simply not something you do for strangers.

Feminists, as we have argued repeatedly throughout this book, should be suspicious of such distinctions; the division between public and private has on the whole been oppressive to women and has been used to keep them out of the public arena. We do, however, have to recognise that such cultural stereotypes are strong. If society views an activity with disgust, only women with few other options will be prepared to do it, and it is precisely those lack of alternatives that can lead to such women being 'exploited'. Nevertheless, we should realise that if such stereotypes can be broken down, surrogacy might be seen in a more positive light as something women might occasionally wish to do for each other, or even for men, as indeed women undoubtedly have done throughout time.

Embryo Research

It was the issue of embryo research that caused the Warnock Committee most trouble, and led its chairperson to write afterwards:

> All the other issues we had to consider seemed relatively trivial compared with this one, concerned as it is with a matter which nobody could deny is of central moral significance, the value of human life.[51]

Although not directly involved in any specific reproductive technology, the issues raised by embryo research are important for us to consider, if only because without past research, reproductive technologies could not have been developed; furthermore, advances in the future will be much slower if research on embryos is not allowed. Moreover, because current techniques of IVF produce spare embryos, some of which may never be transferred to a woman's uterus, they provide the main source of embryos used in research. Questions about embryo research have therefore been explicitly linked to those about reproductive technologies.

The majority position of the Warnock Report was that experimentation should be allowed on embryos for specific research projects, to be licensed by the SLA, up to fourteen days after fertilisation. This particular time limit was derived from the development of the 'primitive streak' which occurs fourteen or fifteen days after fertilisation.[52] The significance of the primitive streak is that its formation is the first time at which cells can be identified which will actually form part of the embryo as opposed to its surrounding environment. And before that point it is possible that twinning can still happen and two or more embryos result or, indeed, that no embryo at all forms. So Warnock drew its cut-off point at the point at which the development of an individual begins, an appropriate point for a committee so careful in general to follow the dictates of rational individualism. But, in practice, its motives for choosing that point were more to do with theological opposition, which tends to be based on the inviolability of the human soul. Logic would lead one to say that the soul cannot have entered the 'pre-embryo' before the appearance of the primitive streak and separation of the embryo proper, unless the soul too can split or disappear if there turns out to be more or less than one embryo there. In practice, of course, such arguments do little to allay religious opposition, which, not being based on rationalist logic, is unlikely to be moved by its exercise.

Further, in line with its logic, most members of the Warnock Committee refused to make a distinction between 'spare' embryos, such as those produced in the course of IVF treatment, and embryos produced specifically for research, arguing that whatever might be permissible to do to one must be acceptable for the other. A minority position, however, supported by two members of the committee, recommended that research should be allowed only on spare embryos, not on embryos specifically brought into existence for research purposes.[53] The Report also unanimously ruled out some specific types of experimentation: in particular, those involving transspecies fertilisation, except in one specific test for male infertility, or the placing of a human embryo in the uterus of another species. They also recommended that the SLA be given the power to prohibit other types of research. The government has gone further than the Warnock Report in this and proposes, whatever other research is or is not allowed, to legislate to ban a number of other types of research procedures, including cloning, genetic manipulation, and ectogenesis, with only parliament, not the SLA, having the power to make exceptions to these prohibitions if new developments make that appropriate.

Three members of the Warnock Committee disagreed with the majority and put in a minority report arguing that all research using human embryos should be banned.[54] The government proposes to allow a free vote of MPs to choose between two legislative clauses: one allowing limited research under licence, the other banning it altogether. This is a completely new way for a government to propose legislation and it has been criticised for effectively ducking what has proved to be the most controversial issue in this whole debate.

It was seen as so important by its critics that it was inevitable that MPs unsympathetic to the rationalist tenor of the Warnock Report should use embryo research as the issue on which to attempt to pre-empt legislation based on Warnock. The first such attempt was made by Enoch Powell in 1985 and various other private members' bills have taken it up since. The very name of Powell's Bill, The Unborn Children (Protection) Bill, set the terms for the subsequent debate and indicated the significance its supporters put on preventing embryo research. The battle lines on this issue were thus drawn along exactly the same lines that they had been over abortion. Roman Catholics, traditionalists and anti-abortionists mobilised strongly in support of Powell, whereas most of the medical profession, women's organisations and other progressives mobilised against. The women's movement saw the Bill both as a way of bringing abortion into question yet again, as its supporters had clearly intended, and as a direct attempt to restrict women's reproductive freedom, by controlling their access to infertility treatment. It was also feared that if passed it would set the tone and institutional framework for subsequent debates on the Warnock Report and other reproductive issues.

The Bill proposed to prevent a human embryo being created, kept or used for any purpose other than enabling a particular child to be born by a particular woman, and that a specific licence would be required from the Secretary of State for Social Services for this in each case. The Bill's implications were appalling not only for embryo research, but also for women seeking IVF treatment. If the Bill had been passed, a government minister, the Secretary of State, would have had to decide which women could receive IVF treatment, without any published guidelines to inform his decisions nor any need to give reasons for any refusal. The medical confidentiality of the women being treated would be destroyed, and the red tape proposed was clearly designed to make IVF even more difficult and slower to obtain than was already the case with waiting lists of up to three years. The Bill would have allowed treatment to continue for a maximum of six months, at a time when the average successful treatment took fourteen months. The treatment would also have been riskier and less effective because all fertilised eggs would have had to be implanted, even those which had no chance of success or were known to be defective. And the situation would never get better as research to improve techniques would have become illegal.

Thus a subsidiary aim of Powell's Bill was to end IVF, without ever saying so explicitly, by making sure that IVF attempts had such a low chance of success that they were not worth the bureaucratic hassle the Bill would impose. It was this aspect of the Bill that gave weight to the claim of its opponents that a subsidiary aim of Powell and his supporters was to control the whole context within which other treatments discussed by Warnock would become law. By setting up such a bureaucratic framework for IVF, it would make it likely that other forms of infertility treatment would be drawn into a similar set-up. By bringing the criminal law further into the reproductive field, the Bill was clearly setting a bad precedent which might encourage further restrictions on women's reproductive freedom.

Powell's Bill was given its second reading by 238 votes to 66, to the profound dismay of the medical establishment, women's organisations and other supporters of the 1967 Abortion Act. However, opposition tactics meant that, like so many private members' Bills, it fell because it ran out of time. Nevertheless, the vote gave encouragement to its supporters who promised to introduce a similar Bill if they won places in the ballot for private members' Bills in subsequent sessions; the Bill did in fact reappear during the next two years but got nowhere near being passed.

In November 1985, in anticipation of further battles, two rival organisations were launched on the same day from the House of Commons. The 'Progress' campaign was sponsored by three MPs, Dafydd Wigley of Plaid Cymru, who had lost two of his own children through a congenital defect; Peter Thurnham, a Conservative who had adopted a severely handicapped child; and Jo Richardson, the Labour Party's most prominent feminist supporter of reproductive rights. The overall aim of 'Progress' was 'to support and protect controlled research into reproduction and prevention of infertility, miscarriage and congenital handicap', and its immediate goal was to prevent parliament passing a Bill outlawing research. The organisation claimed much influential and popular support, including not only the medical establishment but more progressive church leaders, such as the Archbishop of York, and organisations campaigning on behalf of the disabled. They asserted that opposition to research was based on ignorance and, with some justification, that Powell's support had been based on MPs' fear of the organised anti-abortion lobby.

On the same day, 'pro-life' MPs led by the Conservative Sir Bernard Braine launched their campaign 'Progress and Humanity' aiming to 'outlaw the use of the embryonic human being as a guinea pig' and fight for alternative, more ethical research into infertility, genetic disease and other congenital abnormalities. This organisation did not attract much cross-party support. Although forty-four Labour MPs had voted for Powell's Bill, they were heavily censured by the party's conference that year. Indeed, when Tom Clarke, a Labour supporter of Powell, won first place in the ballot for private members' bills the next year, he decided, probably after pressure from his party, not to reintroduce Powell's Bill.

Public opinion seemed at the time to be on the side of 'Progress'. A Marplan poll in May 1985 found 63 per cent in favour of embryo research up to fourteen days to prevent congenital handicap. Although they clearly did not want Powell's Bill, the medical profession was in favour of some legislative guidelines. The Voluntary Licensing Authority, set up by the MRC and RCOG, published its guidelines, which included Warnock's recommended fourteen-day limit, just before the Powell Bill fell. Edwards, the IVF pioneer, argued that fourteen days might be too strict a limit where research might be life-saving, such as into the use of embryonic cells in cancer treatment. Nevertheless, at the same time he pressed for legislation:

> The politicians are letting us down. Someone has got to stick his neck out and make a decision. It's ridiculous having to work without laws. There are no rules, yet we are taking life and death decisions. We need an authority answerable to parliament.[55]

The women's movement in this country has lined up strongly behind those in favour of allowing embryo research.[56] This is quite unlike the position taken in some other countries, such as Australia, where feminists have called for an end to embryo research, questioning both the methods of the research and its aims. They point out that the debates on embryo research rarely consider the women from whose eggs such embryos are obtained.[57] They argue that the power of specialists giving such women their only hope for a child must be so great that women on IVF programmes can effectively be forced to donate 'spare' embryos. And women wishing to be sterilised, the other potential donors of eggs to produce embryos for research, may also be in a weak position to resist pressure to undergo the potential dangers of superovulation for no possible therapeutic benefit to themselves.

These arguments, while of course relevant within the general context of reproductive freedom and sterilisation abuse, do seem somewhat patronising to the women concerned, assuming that they are completely unable to resist pressure. The prevalence of this attitude in Australia among feminists, as opposed to the more liberal attitude to research and infertility treatment in Britain, may reflect the different public profiles of the specialists involved, with the Australian team of Trounson and Wood having taken a much more macho attitude than most British specialists have. More significantly perhaps, Australia has a private health care system, which is one reason why expensive medical techniques such as transplant surgery as well as IVF treatment, whose costs cannot easily be justified within a public health care system, have flourished there. The large profits that can be reaped within such a system make feminists critical of the motives of those who carry out the research needed to perfect these expensive techniques. Researchers have less chance of being seen as benign, and their work less chance of being seen as beneficial, when the financial rewards to themselves are high and depend on the benefits of their research reaching only the very rich.

The other feminist objection, voiced in both countries, has been to the aims of some of this research. In particular the research which looks at the genetic make-up of the embryo again begs a number of questions such as those about the perfect child and our attitudes to the disabled. These are serious questions, but their cutting edge is not so much on the research as the processes of selection and abortion, and it is in our sections on prenatal diagnosis that these specific issues are addressed.

Feminists should be especially wary of accepting the elision of the embryo research issue with that of abortion. It is a position which Powell and his supporters have succeeded in forcing us into in Britain, making the women's movement in Britain much more pro-research than women's movements in other countries. But we should not accept that the status of an embryo in vitro is the same as that of an embryo or fetus that a woman is carrying. In the latter case her personhood is involved, and we do not need to deny the embryo or fetus all consideration in order to retain for her the right of abortion. But for an embryo in vitro, it is only that embryo that is involved, and as the Warnock Report says, it would be most undesirable for women, or anyone else, to hold rights of ownership over embryos. Some feminists rejected Warnock outright because it recommended affording the fetus some protection in law. This seems to us to play into the hands of the anti-abortionists, to accept their terms for the debate rather than making our own; we must show that it is not they but women, as the only possible givers of life to embryos, who have their potential interests at heart.

Access to treatment and the role of the medical profession

The Warnock Report devotes some attention to how decisions should be made as to who should receive infertility treatment and what that treatment should be. Similar questions, though usually turning on a woman's decision not to be pregnant, have been central to all feminist debates about reproductive rights. There are issues both about access to treatment for those who want it and about the nature of the consent that patients are asked to give: how to ensure that they are given sufficient information to be able to decide and given it in a way that does not impose any pressure on them to do what their doctor wants.

When the Warnock Committee started its work in 1982, it took for granted that it should consider whether there were patients who should not be treated for infertility – though one would hardly expect this to be part of the remit of an enquiry into any other branch of medicine. Its report recommended that, in the context of a shortage of available infertility services, where some decision had to be made as to who could be offered treatment, the individual consultant should be left to make that decision. The report claimed that a medical specialist's use of his own judgement about the allocation of such scarce resources was uncontentious when it turned upon issues such as the patient's age, duration of infertility and likelihood that the treatment would be successful. It said, however, that there might be other circumstances in which doctors may also decide that a patient should not be treated for social rather than medical reasons: if such 'treatment would not be in the best interests of the patient, the child that may be born following treatment, or the patient's immediate family'.[58] It declined to suggest any grounds on which such decisions should be made, but did suggest that a patient refused treatment should be entitled to a full account of the reasons for refusal. At no point did the report suggest that somebody other than the medical practitioner might be more appropriate to make such a decision, though it did recognise that this placed a 'heavy burden of responsibility on the individual consultant'.[59]

New reproductive technologies' success stories, at least as they are described in the popular press, turn around their ability to make families complete and happy, and this ideology affects policy makers too. The Warnock Report, as we have noted, almost invariably talks about new reproductive technologies as if they were forms of treatment for *couples*. In doing so it is accepting the idea, current in our society, that children are born to couples. But this approach misses the point that the treatments under discussion are ones that would enable a *woman* to bear a child, and, with the single and rare exception of surrogacy, that the treatment will be done to her. Further, if it is successful, she will be the one to nourish the fetus and give birth to it. One effect of this concentration on couples is to make invisible the problem of infertile women without men to validate their claim to want a child.

The Warnock Report discussed and, in general, ratified under appropriate controls the use of reproductive technologies in the case of cohabiting, heterosexual couples, and only with great reluctance turned their attention to other potential parents such as single people or homosexuals. Although it did not specify any particular group to be unworthy of infertility treatment, the Warnock Committee thought it important to state in their report their own belief 'that as a general rule it is better for children to be born into a two-parent family, with both father and mother'.[60] It used this prejudice to dismiss the view that reproductive technologies could be used to make motherhood possible for women with even less male involvement than that required by sexual intercourse. Indeed, the report's proposal that AID come under the same licensing procedures as other reproductive technologies would make this more difficult. Its recommendations, which effectively enshrine current practice – except for the requirement that reasons for refusal be given – are based on the assumption that treatment should only exceptionally be given to less conventional patients, such as lesbians or other women without a male partner.

Some groups giving evidence to the Committee suggested that people seeking infertility treatment should go through a formal assessment of suitability such as that applied to people wishing to adopt; this would not necessarily rule out single people, who are explicitly provided for in the Children's Act 1975 which covers adoption procedures. Others argued that this would be invidious because people who conceived naturally did not have to be assessed, even though they might have much less well-thought-out attitudes to parenthood than those who had experienced difficulties conceiving. The government's proposals for legislation rejects the idea of any overall statutory procedure to assess suitability. Instead, they recommend that, before granting a licence, the SLA be required to examine a clinic's procedures for deciding whether to offer treatment to particular couples – the government seems simply to assume that only couples will seek treatment. Unlike the Warnock Report, the proposals do not specify that the doctor being consulted should necessarily be the one who makes the decision, but they also make no requirement that people being refused treatment are informed of the reasons.

Thus the relatively benign view of the medical profession that Warnock holds, which would at least allow room for individual variation and the treatment by a progressive doctor of people not falling into the standard categories, is replaced in the government's proposals by a vetting of clinics' selection procedures which is more likely to create uniformity, and close the loopholes through which the unconventional can gain access to infertility treatment. Yet Warnock's proposals, because they rely on the beneficence of the medical profession, also give doctors immense power, and thus fall far short of giving women the right to choose. Feminists, having criticised doctors' willingness to arrogate to themselves the right to decide which women should have abortions, must be similarly concerned that allowing doctors the power to give and withhold infertility treatment could prove dangerous.

In the United States, access is more likely to be an issue fought out in the courts than enshrined in legislation. In Britain, such court cases brought by patients denied treatment are rare and the only one concerning IVF of which we are aware was unsuccessful. A woman, who was told by a Manchester hospital that she and her husband would not make 'suitable parents', lost a case in the High Court to get onto the hospital's IVF programme. In the course of this case, it became clear that all clinics operate some sort of social vetting, discriminating on grounds of age, sexuality, financial security and/or health. Indeed, it was found that NHS clinics, which had waiting lists of up to three years, were the most likely to discriminate; this may be not only because of the pressure of potentially 'worthier' cases waiting to take up available slots, but also because their dependence on public funds might make them more likely to seek social approval.

The Warnock Report did not consider the numerically much more significant discrimination in access to treatment which results from the fact that only one IVF clinic in this country is fully funded by the NHS. Nearly all clinics expect their patients to make some contribution to the costs of their treatment; and the majority of IVF attempts are carried out in private clinics where patients will be expected to pay the full costs. This puts them outside the reach of all but the wealthiest of infertile women and men, and further disadvantages single women and lesbians, who are even less likely than women with male partners to be able to pay for their own treatment. Given the high failure rate of IVF and the large number of attempts usually needed, even in those cases which are successful, a place on a long NHS waiting list may offer no chance at all to an older woman who has already waited a long time before seeking treatment. The government's proposals for legislation nowhere mention the NHS, but that is not so surprising; they were produced at the same time as the government was effectively running down the NHS in favour of privately funded health care.

But the issue of reproductive choice does not only turn on whether or not treatment is actually available. Feminists have in general been critical of the medical profession's handling of women, particularly over the reproductive issues, and have criticised doctors for unsympathetic, imperious attitudes. A fundamental plank of feminism has been the right of women to control their own bodies, an issue which has surfaced most strongly over abortion, rape and domestic violence, but, in some form or other, arises in all doctor–patient encounters. Doctors have been criticised for treating their women patients as incapable of actively participating in their treatment or making decisions, and thus failing to inform women sufficiently of the consequences of treatment or the options available to them. While these criticisms have been levelled at the medical profession's treatment of women in general, they have been felt to apply most strongly to obstetricians and gynaecologists in their treatment of women as actual or potential reproducers.

Both the Warnock Report and the proposed legislation recommend that counselling should be available for all 'couples' contemplating infertility treatment and all potential donors. Such counselling would give information, in a nondirective manner, about the available options; the proposals for legislation list adoption and coming to terms with childlessness as alternatives to be considered to medical intervention. Counsellors would also discuss with couples, where donation is involved, the implications of having a child which is not genetically 'theirs' and with donors the implications, particularly the legal ones, of donation.[61]

Counsellors should be trained and, under the proposed legislation, the SLA will take account of the quality of counselling services when considering whether to grant a licence. The government proposals go further than Warnock and insist that counselling should be distinct from discussions with a doctor about treatment. On the other hand, Warnock devotes some consideration to making sure that the 'couple's' (again) fully informed consent is genuine and suggests that both partners' consent should be obtained, normally in the presence of someone not associated with the performance of the procedures.

Except for the continual reference to couples and the requirement that a woman's partner give consent to procedures which involve her alone, these proposals do reflect some of the concerns expressed by the women's movement about the power doctors have over their patients. However, they are nothing more than best practice procedures for medical decision-making in general and similar practices have not always succeeded in avoiding abuses – with respect to sterilisation, for example. It is the content, not just the form, of counselling to which attention must be given. Here it looks unlikely that an official SLA, given the assumptions we have already seen built into its operation, will be embodying feminist principles.

We should be concerned that women know enough about medical technologies to be aware of their limitations as well as their potential benefits, even though the forms of access which are offered to them, whether the bureaucracy of the NHS and the pressure of its long waiting lists or the expense of the private sector, do not make it easy to insist on, or to know whether one is getting the best information. On the other hand, we must not treat women seeking infertility treatment as perpetual victims, controlling or banning their access to treatment in order that doctors cannot exert their power. Such a view, which implies that women seeking infertility treatment necessarily have their judgement impaired by desperation, focuses its attention too strongly on doctors and the evils one might wish to prevent them doing, and fails to consider the women themselves as human actors, who choose infertility treatment, rightly or wrongly, as a way of taking more, not less, power over their own lives. That women's judgements are influenced by a maternal ideology, of which feminists are critical, does not undercut the argument that they should be left free to make their own choices. None of us can make our minds up free of the influence of social forces, nor indeed should we, for it is in *this society* that we have to carry out the results of our decisions. Counselling cannot by itself change the options that are open to women, but good counselling should provide women with enough insight into their own feelings and the realities of what is being offered to them that their judgements do not produce results very much at variance with their expectations. It is to issues such as these, both the principles feminists need to hold onto in their considering them as well as the actions to which they might lead, to which we now turn in our concluding chapter.

Conclusion: Policy and Politics

In thinking about what to say to conclude this book, we were faced with a dilemma. Our aim was to draw some political implications for feminism out of the preceding discussions of new reproductive technologies. If the feminist principle of 'A Woman's Right to Choose' is inadequate to deal with all the issues that arise out of reproductive technologies, then should we augment it by other feminist principles? Or should we replace it by even more general principles, broad enough to cover all the questions that the development and use of new reproductive technologies give rise to? Or, should we adopt a more pragmatic approach to new developments, weighing the costs and benefits to women of each potential type and use of a technology before pronouncing on it?

Official reports aimed at developing public policy, although not, of course, specifically concerned with feminist issues, have faced a similar difficulty. The Warnock Report poses it as a conflict between the use of rules based on 'moral distinctions, the basic distinctions between right and wrong' and 'utilitarianism . . . which lays down, as the foundation of morality, that an act is right if it benefits more people than it harms, wrong if the balance is the other way'.[1]

There are serious problems with both approaches. The problem with moral absolutes is that they do not take you very far; they tend to result in an insensitive politics which says little about the needs that have given rise to the

Conclusion: Policy and Politics 283

discussion in the first place. In particular, one can have only relatively few feminist principles before they start to conflict with each other. For example, one cannot simultaneously hold to one principle of not allowing any form of sex discrimination and to a second principle of giving all women the right to choose whether or not to have an abortion, including whether to abort a fetus when they find out it is female.

There are also problems with utilitarianism, including that of how to balance the effects on different types of beings. How is harm to an embryo to be measured against harm to a fetus and in turn against harm to a baby, to a child and to an adult? Assuming this measurement problem were solved, which would involve making moral judgements of course, utilitarianism would then allow one to do anything at all if the benefits were great enough. For example, why not transplant the brain cells of a two-year-old if the benefit, in terms of the number of people who could be cured of some terrible disease, is large enough?

The Warnock Committee decided that neither approach could solve the problems it faced. It also decided, however, not to rule out the use of either rules based on moral sentiment or utilitarianism, saying:

> By themselves, then, neither utilitarianism nor a blind obedience to rules could solve the moral dilemmas the Inquiry was faced with. We were bound to have recourse to moral sentiment, to try that is, to sort out what our feelings were, and to justify them. For that a decision is based on sentiment by no means entails that arguments cannot be adduced to support it. Nor are utilitarian arguments based on possible benefits and harm ruled out. It is only that they will not suffice alone.[2]

A similarly eclectic approach informs what we have done. We have decided to give a number of what we hope are useful 'feminist principles' to guide our discussion, but they should not be treated as absolutes. We try to explain both why we hold to them and what their implications are, but we also recognise that they do not tie up all the loose ends and that there may be points at which they conflict, which need resolution.

Similarly, our approach at various points has something in common with utilitarianism, in that we have tended to support procedures which promise clear benefits to some people when we cannot point to any specific harm to others, even when feeling some more nebulous reservations about the morality of doing so. For example, two of the authors felt an immediate revulsion from the process of 'selective reduction' on learning that the bland term meant deliberately puncturing the hearts of some but not all of the fetuses of a multiple pregnancy. But this does not mean that we have come out against it. Rather we have seen it as a technique with potential benefits for some women – both those facing the dangers of an existing multiple pregnancy and those who would wish to make use of techniques which carry the risk of multiple pregnancy.

One reason that we have not condemned particular techniques is that we have taken a relatively libertarian approach, compared with many writers. This is partly because of the long feminist tradition of supporting reproductive rights for women, which in practice has meant supporting a woman's right to choose what is done with her body, even while we recognise the constraints on that choice. Wherever possible, we feel this should be respected. However, we have, at many places in this book, been critical of this approach and do not feel that it alone provides an adequate basis for the sort of reproductive politics that feminism will need to engage in in the future.

In particular it is important to recognise that policy has at least two aspects. One concerns legality, that is whether any of the procedures and techniques that are technically possible should be made illegal. And the second concerns provision: which people should have access to the technologies, how they should be enabled to make use of them, how they should be funded and so on. This may involve the law too, in the prevention of abuses, for example. Currently, there has been much more discussion of the first of these aspects of policy; the Warnock Report is concerned almost entirely with questions of regulation rather than provision or access. But, the counterpart to feminism's relatively libertarian approach, which de-emphasises the role of the law, must be to focus specifically on the second aspect of policy: how whatever techniques and procedures are to be used should be provided, how women are to be able to get access to them and how we should try to influence the directions in which new technologies are developed in the future.

How we see the role of the state is central to any consideration of policy. Do we see the state as potentially beneficial, banning practices only to prevent abuses – but able to be persuaded, within the limits of its budget, to provide what women need? Or should we see it as basically neutral, subject to competing pressures from different interest groups, to which we too must add our voices? Or should we see it as actively inimical to women's interests?

Radical and many socialist feminists have tended to view the state largely as an instrument of male power that works to further the collective interests of those who dominate society. One version of this view sees the state as working directly to favour men's domination over women in, for example, its relative tolerance of domestic violence, and its treatment of married women as the financial dependants of their husbands. A more sophisticated version would see the state involved in perpetuating whatever is the existing social system; in a social system in which women are subordinated to men, the state acts to maintain that subordination. The state, that is, acts to keep the family as a private, financially self-reliant, inviolable unit, so protecting existing relations of reproduction and ensuring that reproduction remains the private responsibility of parents.

But neither view necessarily excludes the possibility of struggle. In both cases women can resist and may at times succeed in forcing the state to act in ways which benefit women. This is the only way, within such frameworks, to interpret women's past successes such as the introduction of child benefit, a benefit paid almost invariably to women, which directly undermines the idea that the family should be financially self-supporting. It is also the only way to interpret the successes of the modern women's movement in challenging existing policies, which mean that women have more reproductive, housing and economic rights than they did twenty years ago, and a little more protection from male violence.

The main way in which feminism has had this effect has been through changing the general climate of opinion, the 'ideology' of the times. The ideas people hold, however, are not independent of the society in which they live; indeed they exist to make partial sense of that society. For just as the state acts to perpetuate the existing social system, so the ideas which appear to make most sense are those which justify the status quo, and thus favour the interests of those who are already dominant. Thus familial ideology, which presents the nuclear family as a natural and harmonious unit, obscures the way women are subordinated within the family, but nevertheless has a strong hold on both men and women in our society as something which appears to be the norm of other people's families if not their own.

Feminists have successfully challenged these ideas: not so successfully that they have evaporated or no longer have a hold on most people, but in such a way that there is more room now for the introduction of alternatives. It is this which has given feminism greater strength and resilience over the past twenty years than the other liberation movements which grew out of the 1960s. We have done so largely by making our issues part of public debate. And it is a measure of our success that so many women, and even some men, feel it necessary to define their positions on a whole range of social issues with respect to feminism. The frequently heard statement 'I am not a feminist but . . .' is actually one of the most hopeful signs.

So in what follows, we have placed some stress on something to which we have given the rather nebulous name 'society' as an arena within which we could hope to have effect. What we mean by this is neither just 'public opinion' nor the 'state' but more the process of getting one to influence the other. We feel that the tasks of feminism must be to both set the agenda for debates on reproductive technologies and ensure that they are kept under public scrutiny. It is through such a process, as well as direct pressure on the state, that we could hope to influence law-making and public provision in a direction that would help women.

The relationship between society and state is not constant, however, and in delineating our principles we recognise that they derive from reproductive politics conducted within a western liberal democracy. That context shapes both the choices women can make and the struggles they engage in. Reproductive choices in other societies will be constrained in other ways; for example, familial ideology may be so much stronger that choosing to be child free is not a viable option for women. Forms of organisation too will be different in the absence of political pluralism. For example, in most Eastern European countries it would be inconceivable, and probably illegal, for a western type of women's health movement to emerge to discuss reproductive issues divorced from state and professional medical control.[3]

Nevertheless, while the context and the extent to which the state controls or limits women's choices may differ from country to country, it is important for feminists everywhere to set the terms of the debate.

Feminist Principles

The principles we discuss below fall roughly into two sorts. The first concern immediate questions about the treatment of individuals. This has been the focus of most reproductive politics in the past and must remain a central concern. These are also perhaps the easier issues for us to think about because we live in a society in which the focus of most politics is on the rights of individuals – even if for women those rights have often proved hard to realise. This means that questions posed in terms of what individuals should or should not be allowed or enabled to do seem the very stuff of politics and the conclusions we come to appear to be ones we might wish to ensure in any society. However, this is somewhat misleading because such issues arise out of the problems of our current society and in practice would impinge very differently in a society in which reproduction was organised differently. For example, in a society in which women were not automatically expected to care for the babies they bore for the next twenty years or so, pregnancy might be experienced quite differently from how it is today. Instead of being primarily the beginning of a long-lasting total commitment, it might be seen more as a nine-month long experience of bodily change and fetal growth and nurturance, with fewer necessary implications beyond that. In such circumstances, not only wanted but unwanted, pregnancies might be experienced very differently from today.

Our principles make a distinction between what we believe the law should prohibit or allow and what we think is in practice desirable. In stating them, we are not saying that we think what is desirable is necessarily easy to achieve: indeed, some of our principles may seem quite utopian. We may feel that all women should have easy access to screening for breast or cervical cancer, for example, although in a health service that is starved of cash that may not be readily attainable. That, however, is no reason not to debate underlying principles: a woman's right to choose has never been particularly easy to attain, yet it must remain a central principle of feminist concern.

Reproductive politics can have another meaning, beyond issues concerning the treatment of individuals. We have stressed, throughout this book, that the effects of new reproductive technologies, and the attitudes people take to them, have to be assessed in the context of the particular sort of society in which we live. And we have been critical of the ways in which the arrangements for reproduction of our society are oppressive to women. *Reproductive politics must also mean finding ways of changing those arrangements.* A first step towards this is to challenge the common assumption that our current way of doing things is natural or inevitable. Moral debates and uncertainties, such as those thrown up by new reproductive technologies, may result in a period of reaction, in which traditional prejudices and ways of doing things are actively reinforced. But equally, the uncertainties can be used to challenge fixed ideas and structures. One aim of feminism must be the latter: to use all possible opportunities to challenge existing relations of reproduction, in so far as they are oppressive to women. The advent of new reproductive technologies provides just such an opportunity, and our second group of feminist principles are concerned with how to make the best use of this opportunity in order to bring down those structures of reproduction that oppress women.

As we have noted at many places in this book, we do not feel that a 'reproductive rights' approach to the issues raised by the new technologies is adequate. In particular, we feel that it tends to make it impossible to discuss the *reasons* why women make particular reproductive decisions. Having said that it is a woman's right to choose seems to leave little room for any further discussion. But, in practice, it is still possible to say that, from a feminist point of view, some reasons for aborting a fetus are good ones, for example, if a woman does not feel ready to be a mother, while others, for example, that she wants only to give her husband a son, are bad ones.

We can hold such opinions without their meaning that we wish to prohibit women from carrying out decisions of which we disapprove. This is for three reasons. The first is that we do not feel our feminist opinions should be forced on others, any more than those of our opponents should. Second, we cannot see any way to prevent such 'bad' decisions being carried out, which do not have the danger of curtailing women's reproductive freedom in much more seriously harmful ways. And finally, we recognise that much greater harm can come of forcing women to bear children they do not want to bear than practically anything else; it is cruel both to the woman and to the child who would be born in such circumstances.

Feminist Principles About the Treatment of Individuals

1. Women should decide whatever is or is not done to their body.

No individual woman nor any group of women, such as the infertile, should be treated as so 'desperate' that they cannot decide for themselves, nor should their decisions be treated as trivial. That choice is never 'free' does not mean there is anyone more appropriate to make it. In particular, doctors should be denied the power to exclude particular women from treatment.

Informed choice has to mean that: doctors should inform, but not decide. The use of counsellors not involved in the treatment is in principle a good idea, but more work is needed to find forms of counselling which are not perceived as directive, but which allow women access to all relevant information. When a woman is deciding about treatment for herself, husband, friends and others should be involved only if the woman actively wants them to be; the decision about any treatment to herself must remain hers alone, though a decision about raising a child within a particular household would have to involve other members too. Clearly the consent of both partners is necessary for treatments that involve both of them; they should be asked to give their consent separately and independently and each should receive individual counselling, with the aim of allowing them to consider their own feelings free, as much as possible, from family as well as outside pressures. To make such decisions, people need to know what the alternatives are and the likely effects of each option; if doctors do not know the answers they should share the extent of their ignorance as well as their knowledge with the people they might treat. But such decisions depend not only on medical factors but on social ones too, and counselling should not be provided only within a strictly 'medical' context. For example, parents should be told what is known about the social effects of raising handicapped children and the range of help available, and be put in touch with support organisations if they want to be.

A pregnancy is the bringing to life of a particular fetus and the knowledge a woman has of its characteristics may well affect her attitude to it. It therefore makes no sense to support abortion on demand for a woman who does not wish to continue to be pregnant, but deny her the abortion if she wants it only once she has discovered that her fetus is disabled, or even female. We may view with dismay a decision to abort a fetus in either or both such cases, but to deny an abortion to a woman who has ceased to wish to carry her fetus would be inhumane, both to the mother and the potential child.

We have to recognise that the availability of prenatal diagnosis makes such abortions more likely and that as a result, more not less stress may be put on women – particularly where pressure comes from others to abort a handicapped fetus or one of the 'wrong' sex. But on balance, we feel that more is to be gained than lost from this. If prenatal diagnosis were to be banned altogether, then some women, who might have chosen not to, will be dedicating their lives to the care of their handicapped children and some children, who might otherwise not have been born, will lead short and painful lives.

We have considered banning the giving of information about the sex of a fetus, but we fear this too holds dangers. If doctors were to be told to withhold this piece of information, we feel they might be encouraged to extend this practice to other areas. Feminists have fought too long against paternalistic attitudes which justify doctors withholding information supposedly for their patients 'own good' to be prepared to countenance any legal enforcement of this practice. Instead, we favour much better counselling of women before they have prenatal diagnosis to help them decide both whether they really want to have it and precisely what information about the results they wish to be given.

In the United States, where every test has to be paid for by parents, directly or through their health insurance, counselling before prenatal testing is much more common, though we do not know the extent to which parents are asked exactly what information they subsequently wish to be given. But in Britain, under the NHS, only certain categories of women are eligible for the more expensive forms of prenatal testing, and the assumption is made fairly automatically that all such women will want to be tested; prior counselling is unknown except in so far as a woman's views on abortion may be canvassed in order to see whether it is 'worth' offering her the test. Indeed, the relatively cheap alpha-fetoprotein blood test is given to pregnant women in most regions of the country without even informing them what it is for. This rigidity of practice and unwillingess to let people decide what happens to them is perhaps the greatest disadvantage of a doctor-dominated, publicly provided health care system over one that would give more voice to consumers; though it is not one that outweighs all its other disadvantages. And there is no intrinsic reason why a publicly funded system should not be made more accountable to consumers' wishes and need for information, without introducing the unfairness of private medicine.

We would therefore advise non-directive counselling of all women so that they seriously consider whether they wish to undergo prenatal diagnosis and precisely which types of results they wish to be told. We would also advise pregnant women not to learn the sex of their child; there is sufficient sex stereotyping that goes on already in our society without it having to start in the womb. Further, the disappointment that can be felt on hearing that a child is the 'wrong' sex can be much more intense when it comes as the only thing that is known about a potential child, rather than as an attribute of a new-born baby whose other real qualities are simultaneously apparent. But we would not impose our views on other women. If they have asked for the tests to be done and wish to know the sex they must be allowed to do so, and if they wish to act on the information they must be allowed to do so too. Any other course will lead to even worse misery, the denial of options which it is dangerous to deny and to acts we have no humane way of preventing.

2. *A pregnant woman is involved in an active process of nurturing an embryo or a fetus; she is producing a baby. She is not just a receptacle in which the fetus or embryo happens to be growing independently. An embryo is only potentially a human being once it is implanted in a woman's womb.*

It is only through the mother's efforts that the potential of an embryo or fetus to develop into a child can be realised. It is not an independent human being since it is not social,[4] nor does it act to shape its environment in any way,[5] two characteristics which have been said to define the difference between fetal and independent human life. On the other hand, it is alive and being grown, by its mother, into a baby; it is a potential baby whose potential cannot be realised without the active involvement of the mother.

Therefore we believe fetuses should be well looked after and mothers given every opportunity to do so, but the language of fetal rights is misleading. Because the mother should be assumed to be the best guardian of a fetus's interests (as she has to be in a day-to-day sense anyway) fetal rights *against* the mother can arise only in exceptional cases.

Those who invoke fetal rights in law tend to do so at specific choice points, such as whether a woman should have a caesarian section for the sake of her baby. Such cases are never clear cut and medical opinion has often proved wrong over such issues; to allow the law to intervene in those relatively rare cases of dispute seems to us a dangerous interference in personal liberty. By casting women in such circumstances as irresponsible – rather than of a different opinion from the medical profession – the much more important continual care a pregnant woman gives her fetus, without which the fetus would never have survived, gets forgotten.

Second, society makes many decisions which, through their effects on pregnant women, deny fetuses many of the advantages that in other circumstances are called 'rights'. We should certainly give some attention to creating an environment which is healthier for fetuses to live in, improving maternal nutrition and banning smoking in all public places, for example. But we should do so, wherever possible, in ways which do not further impose unequal costs on women; for this reason it is preferable, for example, to ensure that all jobs are safe for pregnant women to perform rather than preventing pregnant women, or worse still any woman, from doing particular jobs. But society clearly does not do all it can for fetuses, allowing ill-health and malnutrition of mothers to result in much greater rates of miscarriage, fetal handicap and still-birth in third world countries than in the developed economies of the West. Further, even within the developed world, with the full benefits of modern medical techniques, the survival chances of new-born babies depend critically on the social class of their parents; in Britain perinatal mortality rates of babies born to mothers married to unskilled working class fathers are almost double those of babies with professional parents.[6] Does such a society have the 'right' to impose its will on the bodies of a few individual women for the sake of a possible, though never certain, benefit to their fetuses?

There is no way any embryo can develop into a human being without some woman being willing and able to carry it. This is currently true not only in the narrow sense of what is technologically feasible today, but also in the broader sense of potential developments from known science. To make an artificial placenta would require a qualitative leap in technology that science is nowhere near to reaching at the moment. If such 'ectogenesis' were feasible, this particular set of principles would have to change. But so long as they hold, any time limit on embryo research which refers to a point in time at which the embryo becomes human is meaningless, since any embryo used in research is *never* in practice subsequently implanted. Our view is that potential human life does not exist before implantation and therefore we do not on these grounds rule out experimentation on embryos conceived in vitro, provided any embryo possibly damaged through experimentation is not allowed to become a human life, that is, to be implanted. We do, however, have other criteria to satisfy which are discussed below. This is quite the opposite position from that of our opponents who believe that life has already begun at conception and therefore to deny implantation is to murder, whether or not experiments have already been done; though to be fair, they would not be in favour of doing unsafe experiments in the first place.

There are other issues, besides that of whether an embryo is a human being, which have a bearing on the question of whether embryo research should be allowed and whether a time limit should be imposed. On these questions we feel that a variant of the utilitarian position of assessing the potential benefits to individuals from the results of research over the costs borne by other individuals, particularly in the research, is appropriate. However, this inevitably raises the problem of making inter-personal comparisons, forcing us to weight the harm to one against the benefits to another. In these calculations, the very real costs to the women who have donated the eggs from which the embryos are formed are rarely assessed. But embryos cannot be obtained without subjecting a woman to some discomfort and the risks of surgical intervention. Those costs must be taken account of. They are much more real than any much more speculative potential harm to an embryo.[7]

As far as the embryo goes, in order to avoid the issue of assessing whether the aims of an experiment justify subjecting it to any pain, we suggest that embryos should never be used after the point at which they might be capable of feeling anything at all. Under current British law, animal embryos can be used in experiments at any stage of their development, while human ones cannot. Our view is that, in principle, human embryos are no different from embryos of other mammals.[8] Both should be subject to the same type of protection in law: research on very early embryos cannot cause pain, and should be permitted in principle, while research on later embryos could cause pain and should be controlled.

This means that human embryos should not be used for research beyond the stage at which a nervous system capable of feeling pain develops. This was the position taken by the Royal College of Obstetricians and Gynaecologists who suggested making a time-limit of seventeen days on this basis; as a very conservative estimate of the point at which rudimentary neural development begins.[9] A proper nervous system does not develop until appreciably later. Currently, developing embryos cannot be kept alive to even the fifteen-day limit suggested by Warnock, well before the point at which it is suggested they might be able to feel pain; nor does it look likely that keeping them alive to that point will be possible in the near future. Whatever cut-off point is chosen, not all research that might be carried out before then is equally worthwhile. As with experiments on animals, to question the aims of the embryo research is also valid. We believe some aims, such as the prevention or cure of disease or infertility, and the pursuit of basic scientific knowledge, are rather more worthwhile than others such as the testing of cosmetics, to name a much publicised 'unworthy' use. Assessing the 'worth' of research on animals usually entails making a balance between costs (such as pain caused) and benefits (such as improved medical treatment of people or animals): on this basis, many people feel testing cosmetics on animals to be unwarranted because the benefits to be derived from cosmetics are slight. The costs then outweigh the benefits. Embryo research is somewhat different because there are no costs to the embryo if it does not yet have a nervous system. The costs in the case of embryo research are the effects on the woman from whom the embryo or egg came.

We feel that it is important that the aims of research are assessed and subject to public scrutiny. The current system of local hospital ethics committees is a good idea, but women must have greater representation on such committees. We would also insist that any decisions made by such committees are mandatory, so that researchers cannot simply refuse to change what they do.[10] We would insist, too, that committees make their deliberations fully public and be actively involved in initiating public debate on the issues they have to consider. The denial of secrecy that this would entail can only be to the good; we would hope, for example, that this could put a stop to the dubious practice whereby academic researchers set up companies to sell the results of their research. Commercial pressure for secrecy immediately comes into conflict with the traditions of academic openness and – more importantly – of public accountability.[11]

If we use this approach, the issue of whether only spare embryos should be used or whether it is allowable to create embryos specifically for research becomes straightforward. Neither have the potential for becoming human beings unless they are implanted, and if they are not implanted will never be able to develop to the stage at which they can feel pain. There is no difference from an embryonic point of view in the two cases. However, the way in which they are produced is different and for that reason, under our next principle, we suggest particular safeguards to ensure that donating women are not put under pressure.

3. A fetus or an embryo inside a woman's body is part of her.

Decisions about what is done to a fetus in utero should be made by the woman carrying it. We would make a similar point, though accord it less significance, about gametes – eggs or sperm – while they are still in a human body.

This means that the issue of what can be done with embryos conceived in laboratories, outside a woman's body, is a different issue from what can be done to embryos or fetuses in the womb. In particular, the former has no bearing on the question of abortion. We have to challenge the anti-abortionist position that elides the question of abortion with that of embryo research. To argue that if one worries about experimenting on embryos outside the womb then one should not kill them within, ignores the fact that a fetus in a womb is part of a woman's body. We should not fall prey to that elision and *therefore* automatically defend all forms of research on embryos, as part of our support for abortion rights. The evaluation of experimentation must be on its own merits, and under our proposals above, we would allow experimentation only up to a stage well before that at which an embryo might first be able to feel anything. This stage is much earlier than any time limit for abortions that has ever been proposed. In fact, most women do not even know they are pregnant at that stage, showing how meaningless it is to draw any parallels between the use of embryos for research and the abortion of fetuses.

The control of gametes, embryos and fetuses after removal from a body must be seen as a different question from when they are still in the body. Nevertheless it is clear that women do have feelings about the use of 'their' eggs and embryos, and, of course, about the fate of babies they give birth to. They need some reassurance, but not necessarily control.

In general we favour the view that private property in this context is undesirable; private property can be bought and sold and this inevitably leads to the development of a market and the potential for exploitation. There should therefore be some public agency, rather like an adoption agency, to which people can give their gametes or embryos for donation or research, whenever they are not being directly donated to a particular recipient. This public donation agency would be under full public control and scrutiny and composed of representatives from a wide range of groups with an interest in donation. The agency should see itself as directly accountable to the women and men who use it as well as to the population as a whole. Donations for research purposes would have to be arranged through the agency; this could avoid women being asked to give their eggs or embryos directly to the doctors who treat them, a request that women may find difficult to refuse, particularly if they are currently undergoing treatment as part of IVF.[12] This does not mean that donors cannot express their wishes as to what happens to their gametes or embryos, or learn the results of research which they have made possible, but that is different from having the full control we would expect someone to have of a part of their own body or the rights of disposal people have over private property.

The public donation agency should, in particular, work to ensure that the interests of women as potential donors of eggs and embryos are protected fully. Egg donation is a much more complex and risky procedure than donating sperm; eggs will therefore always be in short supply and it will be particularly important to ensure that women are not put under any pressure to donate. Further, women should not be subjected to any medical treatments that might facilitate 'donation' indirectly without their explicit consent. They should not, for example, be given higher doses of hormones than necessary in order to make them produce surplus eggs for research or donation. The donation agency should provide counselling to ensure that women themselves make any decisions about donation without coercion.

Denying individuals the right of ownership in gametes or embryos once they are no longer in a human body would prevent a market in them developing and avoid the exploitative relations that market pressures stand to impose. We would ideally envisage an entirely free system, rather like the blood transfusion service, although we do recognise that egg and embryo donation require rather more of a woman than giving blood. Of course, the donation agency would have to be part of a free health service, to protect the health of donating women.

The British blood transfusion service does show some of the advantages of a free medical donation system over one where 'donors' are paid. Payment can provide an incentive for donors to disguise the fact that they may be carriers of a disease; it is the use of imported blood that had been collected for payment which is thought to have led to the spread of Aids among haemophiliacs even in Britain. Further, if payments are made, there is an incentive to evade checks on how frequently a person has given blood and the poor may risk their own health in the process.

Similar disadvantages, we believe, would attend any paid system whereby reproductive tissue was donated. If, for example, women could 'donate' aborted fetuses for research in exchange for payment, there is considerable danger that women might be pressurised into conceiving and then aborting – procedures that impose risks to their health. In particular, we see no reason why sperm donors should be paid, as they usually are in most countries today; sperm donation is much the easiest form of donation under consideration.

In France, there is a nationally co-ordinated network of sperm banks, called the Centre d'Etudes et de Conservation de Sperme (CECOS). CECOS organises sperm donation throughout the country and encourages men to see 'donation as an act that affirms their membership of society at large, a gift that acknowledges the needs of some in the community'.[13] It wraps this up in a familial ideology in which couples give sperm to other couples; indeed only married donors are accepted. The aim of this is to project an image of sperm donation as a principled, public spirited act. This is quite unlike the way it is seen in most other cultures where it is just a clandestine, inconsequential way in which medical students make a bit of extra money. We would see our public donation agency operating in some ways like CECOS, though without the familial ideology. In particular, we would see our agency as actively involved in promoting a positive image of donation and in encouraging debate.

Some feminists have argued against any form of state intervention in reproductive processes, fearing that the involvement of a male-dominated state can only be to women's detriment. While sympathetic to this view, we feel, however, that the dangers of total non-regulation, the development of a market and the exploitative relations that entails, are much more serious. Although the odds may be stacked against us, we see the state, as we have argued above, as a site for feminist struggle in which some battles can be won. The control of our public donation agency and the ideology under which it operates may be one such battle. Again adoption agencies may provide an apt analogy. They work reasonably well, despite some reservations about their procedures; their tendency to insist that adoptive parents are young, heterosexual and married is perhaps the most worrying from a feminist point of view. But if adoption was to be seen as a feminist issue, and feminists became involved in contesting adoption procedures, these could be changed for the better. Further, no feminist has suggested that it would be preferable to have a totally unregulated system, in which babies were effectively private property and a market in children was allowed to develop.

On the issue of anonymity of donation, we do not think there should be any hard and fast rules. We do not share the desire of officialdom to normalise all the families created by donation by denying the donor an identity. On the other hand, we do recognise that, living as we do within a society in which the infertile mostly wish to create just such a 'normal' family for themselves, we should not deny them that chance. We therefore feel that the public donation agency should be prepared both to cater for anonymous donation, and to make possible a variety of forms of greater involvement by known donors, subject to clear guidelines to protect the rights of all parties, where this was desired by both donor and recipient. In particular we do not wish to discourage women from having the opportunity of helping each other, either in general or a particular friend. In the latter case, the public donation agency might be involved in counselling and making subsequent legal arrangements, but not in actually arranging the donation.

In general, we are sympathetic to the idea of self-insemination by women, but we do recognise that it has its dangers. We do not agree with the government's legislative proposals which insist that all artificial insemination should be officially regulated. But, in order to avoid the risk of disease and to retain access to any important medical history of donors, we would prefer women to use our public donation agency, especially when they are trying to have anonymous donation. In current conditions many women may feel disinclined to use any public agency, fearing a loss of control and possible discrimination. To counteract this valid fear the public donation agency must be open equally to all women who want to use it.

4. Enabling people to carry out their reproductive choices should be an important aim of public policy.

We do not use the language of rights here because, as soon as this is extended beyond a right to be able to terminate an unwanted pregnancy, it clearly cannot be met in full. No state can give a woman the right to bear a child, and although it could guarantee all women the 'right' to medical consultation and treatment for infertility, such a right could not be absolute unless the state was prepared to underwrite unlimited resources to this end.

Nevertheless, we believe that such things are worth spending public money on. To dismiss the desire of women and men to be parents as just one potentially unfulfilled desire among many is to fail to recognise the importance of reproduction to society, and the importance it plays in the lives of individuals. We may wish to combat a tendency to place too much importance on reproduction at a personal level, particularly when women fail to see themselves as anything more than potential mothers. But in any society, reproduction will be essential for the perpetuation of that society and should be accorded at least as much importance as those 'productive' tasks that we have less difficulty valuing. One reason for the non-recognition of the importance of reproductive work to society is that it is done by women; it is perhaps the most telling example of how the sexual division of labour immediately renders less important whatever is put on the female side of the divide.

But, it is important that whatever resources are devoted to giving women reproductive choices should be spent efficiently to help as many women as possible. This means that money spent on combating infertility would be best spent on preventative programmes. These would involve, among other measures, trying to check the spread of infections which have rendered women and men infertile, and making access to clinics for their treatment easier and less intimidating so that women, in particular, who may have less obvious symptoms and more to fear from unsympathetic attitudes, receive early and fast treatment.

Some infertility is caused by previous medical interventions, so prevention includes ensuring that all treatments are absolutely necessary and done as safely as possible. Abortions, for instance, should be carried out in the safest and most hygienic circumstances and as early as possible, which present legal requirements make impossible. If the large sums that are spent on high-tech treatment for the few were spent on such preventative programmes, the number of men and women that could be prevented from becoming infertile would be much greater than the number that are currently helped by reproductive technologies.

But however much was spent on prevention, there would still be some people who would seek infertility treatment. We do not feel it would be appropriate to offer them nothing. We therefore think that there should be some provision of infertility treatment, including reproductive technologies. It is also important that some research continues in these areas, because they may have spin-offs which can help far more people.

For prenatal diagnosis, public funds are more likely to be forthcoming, since any government which contributes at all to the care of the handicapped will save money by preventing the birth of babies with congenital diseases. But on these grounds alone, not all women would be offered all the tests, only those whose risk of carrying an affected fetus is sufficiently high that money will be saved by making the test available, rather than letting such fetuses be born. We agree that all such women should be offered prenatal testing, but, in line with the above principle, we believe that more should be spent on prenatal diagnosis than would be justified on a purely cost-saving basis. In particular, this means providing women of all social groups with equal access to clinics and counselling. There should, for example, be just as many clinics offering genetic counselling for sickle cell disease as there are for cystic fibrosis.

Women of lower risk should be offered the chance of prenatal testing too, as an aspect of reproductive choice, though we do not expect all women to take up such an offer; even among those who would like to know the results many may decide that the risks of the procedure are not worth it in their case. Further, we think it important that whatever tests are offered to women are offered whatever her views on abortion, and no woman should be asked to agree to an abortion in order to get a test.

5. All women should have access to reproductive technologies on the same terms.

No woman or man should be denied infertility treatment by prejudice: for example, beliefs that there are already enough black babies born, or that lesbians do not make good parents. Discrimination in treatment on grounds of colour, sexual preference, marital status or disability should be made illegal. If people receiving infertility treatment subsequently prove bad parents they can be treated like any others and the children rescued, if necessary, from an unsatisfactory situation. Although this may sound callous with respect to the children, there is no way of avoiding such situations, which may occur whatever vetting procedures are adopted. There is no reason at all to allow doctors, who have no training in the matter, to act as exceptionally prescient social workers and make their own judgements as to who will and who will not be a good parent. On the other hand, we do see a role for independent, non-directive counsellors, who should enable people coming for treatment to think through their wishes for children which, given the lengthy experience of infertility treatment, may have become somewhat divorced from the everyday realities of being a parent. But the final decision whether to go for treatment or not must be that of the person or couple who would receive it.

This is the very opposite of the government's proposals which insist that a clinic's licence should depend on it having good vetting procedures. In our view any clinic found to have vetting procedures should be closed down. Further, a refusal to treat should be able to be challenged in the courts; this would provide a further safeguard against clinics practising unlawful discrimination by using unsubstantiated medical grounds to deny people treatment.

There is a second problem about ensuring equal access which is much more difficult to solve even in theory. In any country which allows private medical care, the most consistent form of discrimination practised is by income. Anyone who can pay can jump queues in the National Health Service, and infertile couples who pay can attempt IVF more quickly and more frequently, though not necessarily with any greater success each time, than people who cannot. In general, we would favour a totally public health care system, in which private practice was made illegal for anyone *eligible* to practise within the health service, whether or not they actually did so.

But we are far from having the power to abolish private medicine. While private clinics remain, we would insist that they should have to take anyone who comes to them for treatment and charge a sliding scale of fees, dependent on patients' income, which would go down to zero for those on low enough incomes. If such an insistence meant a few of the smaller clinics closed down, we do not think this would be such a great loss; their success rates are rather low, anyway.[14] The larger clinics could clearly survive such practices, their international reputations would allow them to put up their fees considerably to the very rich. If ultimately they found operating such a system too much of a handicap, they could perhaps offer themselves to the National Health Service.

All this does imply some form of regulation, but we would want to see this done by a body more accountable to the people, and in particular to the women who are most crucially affected by their decisions, than the government's proposed Statutory Licensing Authority. The government's SLA was designed to regulate the behaviour of a number of independent, mostly private, clinics. We would rather see a more organic system, a network of publicly funded clinics, which could ensure that existing techniques were being provided on a scale to meet demand.

To ensure accountability and effective representation we would insist that the authority has a substantial majority of women members, some of whom should have had problems with their own fertility. In order to monitor discrimination properly we would also like to see an effective representation of people with disabilities, ethnic minorities, lesbians and gay men on the authority. At present, this seems somewhat over-optimistic. In the meantime, while people with views like ours have little direct effect on current government thinking, perhaps the best way we can hope to influence policy is through arguing for the representation of as many non-establishment groups as possible on such a board and through continual monitoring by feminist groups of its activities.

Principles Which Challenge Existing Relations of Reproduction

We now move on to consider a second set of principles, ones which also say something about how we would like to see new reproductive technologies used, but which have the further aim of helping to transform the way reproduction is organised in our society. Few, if any, of these principles are new or controversial within feminism. They have won widespread support before in other contexts. However, their application to the issues of this book may result in conclusions that are different to those of some other feminist writing on reproductive technologies.

1. *Change that breaks down the identification of social parenting with biological processes should be encouraged.*

This is for two reasons. First, because it is important for women to be able to show that there is nothing natural or necessary about current social arrangements concerning reproduction. New reproductive technologies involving donation will reinforce the message, which successful adoption already carries, that social parents do not need to be biological ones. And this should enable one to question the more oppressive aspects of 'normal' reproduction within the nuclear family, in which women, largely in isolation, rear children. In particular, it should lay to rest the notion that child-rearing is just a natural instinct of women brought about by a genetic connection, a necessary sequel to the experience of pregnancy and childbirth, rather than real work which other people can undertake too.

Artificial techniques for overcoming fertility are not to be rejected just because they are unnatural, or because they involve people other than biological parents. Women have far more to lose from an insistence that our current social arrangements are natural than from questioning them. For that reason, we have stressed arrangements for donation in our proposals above. We feel that it is around these types of arrangements, which involve breaking down the isolation of nuclear families and people helping each other across familial boundaries, that there is most chance of a specifically feminist input being made to discussions on new reproductive technologies and of those discussions leading to a rethinking of current practices.

But the implications of this go far beyond those cases where technology is used. In particular, we believe that feminists should pay more attention to the politics of adoption and fostering. We would like to enable more women to consider flexible arrangements over reproduction, so we would like to see the stigma that currently attaches to women who choose to give up their children removed. Women should not have to be committed from the moment of conception, or the moment of choosing not to have an abortion, to responsibility for a child for the next twenty years or so. In particular, we suggest that birth should be seen as a real choice point where women are enabled to consider the option of not continuing to be the one to care for the child they have nourished in their womb. Men have always had the possibility of escaping from the care of the children they biologically father. We have tended to see that as irresponsibility, as it usually is when the responsibility is then just dumped on a woman. But if everyone felt they had a choice and knew that their children would still be well looked after, children on the whole would be cared for more, not less, responsibly and women would be enabled to have more genuine reproductive choices.

Indeed, if the giving up of children for adoption were more acceptable, so that women did not see it only as a last resort following an unwanted pregnancy, then some women might think of helping others, by bearing a child for them. We might even find that there were women who had babies because they enjoyed pregnancy, or wanted to experience it for the first time, without being sure that they necessarily wished to devote the next twenty years to raising a child. We feel that in this context, the abortion decision would, in practice, be freer; instead of women seeing the alternatives as being either to have an abortion or to make a long-term commitment to looking after a child, we could add a third possibility, to experience pregnancy and childbirth and then let someone else raise the child.

We would favour allowing a variety of social arrangements

for adoption, from the current one of severing all connection with the biological mother to ones that enabled more involvement. But whatever types of arrangements were made would have to be chosen by all parties, and we recognise that in current circumstances, most adoptive parents would probably prefer to be able to create a similar sort of nuclear family to that chosen by most biological parents. In this, as in other considerations, we should not expect individuals, particularly those in unfortunate circumstances, to right the wrongs of society. For this reason too, we do not accept the argument that while there are children who cannot be placed for adoption, because they are too old or suffer from some disability, we should not be concerned about the difficulties of parents wishing to raise a healthy baby.

2. *The experiences of childbearing and rearing should be given more weight than that of providing a man or a woman with a child to whom they are genetically related.*

If society moves in the direction we would like to see, then genetic connections will seem less important, and social parenting more so. But even today, it seems to be men more than women who are most concerned to have a genetic connection with the children they raise. This is not surprising, for given the minimal social parenting role that society expects of men, a genetic connection is all they may feel they have with their children, while women know they have much more. Thus women on IVF programmes are more likely to be prepared to consider adoption than their partners. Some women are even going through the rigours of IVF mainly because their husbands will not consider adoption, while a few are there because not they, but their partners, have a fertility problem – producing too few sperm for normal fertilisation to work – and have presumably rejected AID as a solution.

Feminists may not approve of the way in which men influence women's choices – particularly when women are thus exposed to the risks and trauma of surgical intervention simply to provide a husband with his own genetic progeny. But that is not an argument for denying an individual woman the right to choose what is done to her body. Until existing relations of reproduction change, some women are going to make choices that we do not like.

We recognise that in current conditions genetic links can seem important to both men and women and, again, we do not wish to deny to the infertile chances that are available to the fertile. Techniques whose main purpose is to further a genetic connection should therefore still be made available, at least in the short term, provided women's rights to make their own choices are protected, and the following principle is adhered to.

3. Individuals, not couples, should be the focus of infertility treatment.

A tendency to blur what is going on arises from the way policymakers and doctors talk of a 'couple' being treated for infertility. In practice, the medical cause of infertility has about an equal chance of lying with the man or with the woman or being to do with some interaction between the two of them. However, both conventional treatment and new reproductive technologies require much more of women than of men, so it is the woman who must think particularly hard whether for her it is worth going through with treatment. In most cases, those where the medical problem lies with the man or in the interaction between the two partners, she could avoid all the problems of treatment by using donated sperm or choosing another partner.

We therefore would argue that when couples request treatment, counselling for both partners should include information about their chances of successful reproduction with donated genetic material and/or other partners. While we believe that counselling should be non-directive and should support women's rights to make independent choices, counselling should do more than simply present information about donated genetic material as a solution to a biological problem. Ideally, such counselling should enable people to understand better the social context of rearing children, so that they can consider all options including adoption or using donated material.

It is questionable whether enabling a fertile woman to bear the child of her sub-fertile husband should be considered a 'medical' aim at all – since the patient whose infertility is 'cured' is the man, but it is the woman who has to bear the trauma of surgical intervention. We need to have strict guidelines laid down for cases like these, at least as stringent as those for the circumstances in which healthy volunteers can be used to test a drug to cure other people. Treating infertility as a couple's problem can easily obscure these issues.

Donation, or even choosing another partner, can also be a solution to the problem of inherited genetic diseases. If the man is the carrier of a dominant gene, such as that for Huntington's disease, or both partners are carriers of recessive genes, for genetic diseases such as thalassaemia, sickle-cell anaemia or Tay-Sachs disease, then AID can be a way to avoid the trauma of prenatal testing and late abortions. It should not be assumed that women necessarily have to bear their partner's child, nor that they all would think doing so important enough to risk genetic problems, if the alternative of AID were put to them. Similarly, if the woman is the carrier of the dominant gene, egg donation could be considered as a way to avoid prenatal testing, though this is a procedure which must be at least as stressful for most women as a late abortion (and is, of course, stressful for both the donor and the recipient). These considerations also point, of course, to the desirability of making counselling available to fertile men and women before conception.

4. *We should not allow reproductive technologies to erode the freedoms that current reproductive arrangements allow.*

Not everything about current reproductive arrangements is terrible. Pregnancy, childbirth and raising children provide some women with the experiences they value most highly in their lives. That this can so often be the case is another consequence of the separation of the public and the private, whose deleterious effects we criticised earlier. Reproduction, by being located so clearly in the private, is also free of some of the worst aspects of the public sphere, in particular, the one-dimensional, self-interest of economic life. If people behaved in their private lives as they do in the marketplace, nobody would ever get involved in bringing up children. For to raise children demands a great deal of self-sacrifice for little, if any, personal gain, though the rewards, in quite a different sense, can be immense. To preserve those private satisfactions, it is important to keep the morals of the marketplace out of reproduction, which is not, of course, to say that women do not deserve economic recognition for the work they do in bringing up children.

This means that the issue of surrogacy has caused us some problems. On the one hand, we do not see why women should not be enabled to help each other in this way, nor do we have problems with the notion of a woman choosing, rather than being forced by adverse circumstances, to give up a child she has given birth to. It is the idea of a surrogacy *contract* that worries us. For this can only be designed to restrict the experience of pregnancy. Edward Yoxen notes how surrogate mothers under contract are often quoted as talking about having to 'work' at their feelings, and this 'willed alienation' is what worries him most because it 'renders yet another area of our lives into mere work'.[15] Even if not all surrogate mothers have these problems, the point still holds that a surrogacy contract introduces, into one of the few areas which have remained free of it, the coercion of having a contract of exchange to fulfil.

We would propose our public donation agency as the appropriate body to make 'surrogacy' arrangements, assuming all the safeguards we noted above. But we would envisage surrogacy arrangements taking a different form from what is meant by the term today; indeed we do not like the term much either. Instead, we would see surrogacy as another form of donation, in this case of the time and physical effort of carrying a baby. We would therefore propose that the agency looks for women who are in principle willing to bear children for other people, but imposes no contractual obligation on them and, in turn, makes no promises to the people who wish to raise the child. In practice, unless genetic material from the would-be parent or parents is used, this is no different from encouraging women who choose to have babies for adoption, mentioned above. As with adoption, it would be essential that safeguards were built into arrangements, to prevent women from being coerced. Coercion need not be directly linked to financial gain; women should be subject to no pressure to comply with what may be perceived by others as an unwritten obligation.

We would put a relatively low priority on providing genetic connections and if this cannot be done without leading to the problems of contracts, as particular parents await the delivery of particular children, then we feel that such arrangements, which are in practice the crux of what is normally meant by 'surrogacy', must be abandoned.

5. Public debate about reproductive technologies should be encouraged.

The secrecy which surrounds reproductive problems at the moment helps nobody; infertility, miscarriages, abortions and other reproductive problems should not be something people feel that they have to hide. We should aim to break the conspiracy, fuelled by familial ideology, that reproduction is normally a smooth process with happy results. The effect of this is to marginalise women for whom things go wrong and make their unhappiness more intense.

Public debate can also help break down the isolation of women having to make difficult reproductive decisions on their own, such as whether or not to abort a handicapped fetus. If a woman knows that others have faced similar problems and is familiar with the arguments on both sides, she may find the burden of choice and responsibility less hard to bear. She may also be less subject to immediate family pressures, if she has the weight of other women's experiences to call on.

Furthermore, it is through public debate that we have most chance of being able to influence practices surrounding reproduction, including reproductive technologies, in a feminist direction. We must keep reproductive technologies on our political agendas, to ensure that the issues that arise get full and continuing public discussion. Reproduction remains one of the most privatised activities in our society and to question its most oppressive aspects, by making reproductive technologies a matter of public debate, can only be to the good. We must do so if we wish to have any hope of building a society in which our feminist principles are taken as common sense.

6. Women should have more control over future developments in reproductive technology.

If developments in reproductive technology are truly to serve women's needs, then we must have greater control over their development. In part, we could gain greater control if there were more women working in science and technology. But that alone would not be enough: as feminists have often lamented, bringing more women into a particular sphere does not necessarily change its direction.

What is more important, and more fundamental, is that science and technology in general are made much more publicly accountable, so that women's needs are met. As we saw in Chapter Two, science and technology are far from being publicly accountable; moreover, the direction of research is governed far more by the policies of funding bodies (and by prevailing ideologies) than it is by actual social needs. Science has to become not only more accountable, but much more sensitive to *public* debate in all areas where ethical issues are raised; these include such issues as the ethics of using animals, human volunteers or embryos in experiments, as well as the more general ethical issues raised by reproductive technologies.

It is important, too, that women are more involved in the design of any new technology intended to intervene in reproduction. If devices are to be used *on* women's bodies (such as ultrasound devices), then women are the people best suited to designing them and assessing their impact. The design of a technology is not, of course, independent of the social context in which it occurs; so even if women are involved, it may still not be ideal for all women. Nevertheless, to introduce more women into the design process would undoubtedly be an improvement.

We must also challenge science policy more broadly. Science policy makers are rarely women, and feminist questions are hardly ever raised in relation to national science policy. It is important for women that we gain more control over policy issues, including the fundamental questions of what research should be encouraged or funded. This is vital whether feminists decide to challenge only some of the new developments, or feel that all new reproductive technologies pose a threat to women: either way we will have to tackle state policy.

Among other things, this means ensuring that research does relate to women's needs, and to the needs of all women equally. So, for example, we should not encourage research into genetic diseases that particularly affect the white population if that means less is spent on research into diseases affecting other, less powerful, social groups. Having more control over science policy should also include the possibility of banning a particular kind of research if there is evidence that it will work against women's interests.

If women are to gain more control over the future development of reproductive technologies, then we must demand that research into reproduction and possible means of intervention become more sensitive to what women want; unless and until ectogenesis becomes available, reproduction cannot occur without women's bodies and on that basis we should insist on playing a central part in all decision processes. To change existing relations of reproduction means changing a situation in which women are always the passive objects of scientific scrutiny. What that means is nothing less than challenging the monolithic power of science itself.

So these are our principles and their implications. We have not felt it necessary to take a position on all the fine details of legal debates over donation and rights – these are mainly concerned with preserving the status quo, its property relations, the rights of fathers and putting children into families. We are in favour of breaking down the uniformity of family relations and so cannot hope to sort out all the loose ends that might be thrown up; if people are not to be forced into inappropriate legal categories a little untidiness in this area must be expected.

Some of our suggestions are undoubtedly optimistic; arguing for a system of free clinics and counselling services while the National Health Service is under attack may even seem perverse. But the advent of the new reproductive technologies poses feminists with many challenges; however we view particular technologies, we have to meet those challenges. Some of our principles have implications that suggest sites for feminist struggle – for instance, the principle that access to available technologies should be on equal terms to all women. Others present us with an even more substantial challenge, such as breaking down the link between biological and social parenting, or challenging the power of science. But if we want to prevent new developments in reproductive technology from being used to erode those rights that we do have, then those challenges are essential.

Notes

Introduction

1. National Opinion Polls cited by M. Simms, 'Legal abortion in Great Britain' in H. Homans (ed.) *The Sexual Politics of Reproduction*, Gower, Aldershot, 1985, p 94.
2. The Women's Reproductive Rights Campaign is currently run from the York Women's Centre, 11 Holgate Road, York YO2 4AA.
3. The Women's Health and Reproductive Rights Information Centre publishes a quarterly newsletter and a wealth of information sheets on reproductive technologies and other reproductive and health issues which can be obtained from WHRRIC, 52 Featherstone Street, London EC1Y 8RT.
4. Warnock Committee, *Report of the Committee of Inquiry into Human Fertilisation and Embryology*, Cmnd 9314, HMSO, London, 1984.

1. Reproductive Freedom, Technology and Society

1. See, for example, Steven Goldberg, *The Inevitability of Patriarchy*, Temple Smith, London, 1977 for a sociobiological account that is totally explicit about its intentions.
2. Central Statistical Office, *Social Trends*, 18, HMSO, London, 1988, p 48.
3. Even of women born in 1920, 21 per cent had not had children in 1985, *Social Trends*, loc.cit.
4. See N. Chodorow, *The Reproduction of Mothering*, University of

California Press, Berkeley, 1978 and D. Dinnerstein, *The Rocking of the Cradle*, Souvenir Press, London, 1978.
5. Some such views are expressed in terms that are in our view insulting to infertile women. For example, one prominent opponent of reproductive technologies and founder member of FINRRAGE writes that: 'Women, motivated by an intense life crisis over infertility, are manipulated by this situation ['their "need" (social or otherwise) to have babies'] into full and total support of any technique which will produce those desired children, without consideration of the implications of doing so for women as a social group', R. Rowland, 'Motherhood, patriarchal power, alienation and the issue of "choice" in sex preselection' in Corea et al (eds.) *Man-Made Women*, Hutchinson, London, 1985, p 75.
6. V. Roggencamp, 'Abortion of a special kind' in R. Arditti, R. D. Klein and S. Minden (eds.), *Test-tube Women: What Future for Motherhood?*, Pandora, London, 1984 and M. Kishwar, 'The continuing deficit of women in India and the impact of amniocentesis' in G. Corea et al, *Man-made Women: How New Reproductive Technologies Affect Women*, Hutchinson, London, 1985.
7. B. Katz Rothman, *The Tentative Pregnancy*, Penguin, New York, 1987, p 180.
8. W. Farrant, 'Who's for amniocentesis? The politics of prenatal screening' in H. Homans (ed.) *The Sexual Politics of Reproduction*, Gower, Aldershot, 1985.
9. B. Hoskins and H. Holmes, 'Technology and prenatal femicide' in Arditti, Klein and Minden, op.cit.
10. S. Hillier, 'Women and population control in China: issues of sexuality, power and control', *Feminist Review*, 29, 1988.
11. R. Steinbacher, 'Sex preselection: from here to fraternity' in C. Gould (ed.) *Beyond Domination: New Perspectives on Women and Philosophy*, Rowman and Allanheld, Towota NJ, 1984.
12. T. Powledge, 'Unnatural selection: on choosing children's sex' in H. Holmes, B. Hoskins and M. Gross (eds.), *The Custom-Made Child? Women-Centered Perspectives*, Humana Press, Clifton NJ, 1981 and Rothman op.cit.
13. Rothman, op.cit., pp 100–1.
14. Rothman, op.cit., p 11.
15. See, for example, Catherine Hall, 'The butcher, the baker, the

candlestickmaker: the shop and the family in the Industrial Revolution' and 'The home turned upside down? the working-class family in cotton textiles 1780–1850', both in E. Whitelegg et al (eds.) *The Changing Experience of Women*, Martin Robertson, Oxford, 1982.
16. M. O'Brien, *The Politics of Reproduction*, Routledge & Kegan Paul, London, 1981.
17. M. Stanworth, 'The deconstruction of motherhood', in M. Stanworth (ed.) *Reproductive Technologies*, Polity, Cambridge, 1987, pp 23–4.
18. In 1985 and 1986, 72 per cent, the highest proportion ever of divorces were granted to wives: *Social Trends*, op.cit., p 43.
19. From over 10,000 in 1971, the number of adoptions of children under two years old fell more than 80 per cent to just over 2,000 in 1986, *Social Trends*, op.cit., p 48.
20. A woman treated in one of the larger IVF centres has a 1 in 5 chance of giving birth to a live baby: *The Third Report of the Voluntary Licensing Authority for Human In Vitro Fertilisation and Embryology*, Medical Research Council, London, 1988.
21. This argument has been put to one of the authors most forcefully by a colleague and is, we suspect, not an uncommon view. However, we cannot find any written reference to it, even in the most enthusiastic population control literature.
22. The Chinese however now seem to think that their one child policy was a failure, but this may be more of an indication of a change of ideology about reproductive freedom than a claim that it did not actually reduce the birth rate among some groups of the population. S. Hillier, op.cit., p 106.
23. A survey of consultant obstetricians found that three-quarters of respondents said they generally require women to agree to termination of an affected pregnancy before proceeding to amniocentesis, Farrant, op.cit., p 113.

2. Science, Technology and Nature: Women's Friends or Foes?

1. Shulamith Firestone, *The Dialectic of Sex*, Jonathan Cape, London, 1971, p 19.
2. Leon Kass, *Toward a More Natural Science: Biology and Human Affairs*, The Free Press, New York, 1985. pp 2–3.
3. Ibid., p 33.

4. Ibid., p 347.
5. See, for example, Penelope Brown and Ludmilla Jordanova, 'Oppressive dichotomies: the nature/culture debate'. In: *Women in Society: Interdisciplinary Essays*, Cambridge Women's Studies Group (eds), 1981, Virago, London.
6. For a discussion of feminism in relation to technological change see, for example, Jan Zimmerman, *Once Upon the Future*, Pandora, London, 1986; Cynthia Cockburn, *Machinery of Dominance*, Pluto, London, 1985; and Wendy Faulkner and Erik Arnold (eds), *Smothered by Invention*, Pluto, London, 1985.
7. Robert Winston, *Infertility: A Sympathetic Approach*, Macdonald Optima, London, 1987, p 169.
8. Rev. Francis Harman, cited in Edward Yoxen, *Unnatural Selection: Coming to Terms with the New Genetics*, Heinemann, London, 1986, p 63.
9. Italics in original. Cockburn, op.cit., 1985, p 255.
10. For criticism of this view, see, for example, Lynda Birke, *Women, Feminism and Biology*, Wheatsheaf, Brighton, 1986.

3. The Medicalisation of Reproduction: Justifications and Assumptions

1. Naomi Pfeffer and Anne Woollett, *The Experience of Infertility*, Virago, London, 1983, p 22.
2. Christine Crowe, '"Women want it": *in-vitro* fertilization and women's motivations for participation'. In: *Made to Order: The Myth of Reproductive and Genetic Progress*, Patricia Spallone and Deborah Lynn Steinberg (eds), Pergamon, Oxford, 1987.
3. Ibid. p 90.
4. Ann Oakley, 'From walking wombs to test-tube babies'. In: *Reproductive Technologies*, Michelle Stanworth (ed.), Polity, London, 1987, pp 54–5.
5. Crowe, op.cit. p 93.
6. Detailed research on, for example, Islamic law and abortion is, however, lacking: see Janet Black & Sophie Laws, *Living with Sickle Cell Disease*, Report produced for the East London Branch of the Sickle Cell Society, 1986, pp 271–2.
7. M. G. R. Hull, 'Infertility: nature and extent of the problem'. In: *Human Embryo Research – Yes or No?*, The Ciba Foundation, Tavistock, London, 1986, p 25.
8. Mary Warnock, *A Question of Life*, Blackwell, Oxford, 1985, p 13.

9. W. Cates, T. M. M. Farley and P. J. Rowe, 'Worldwide patterns of infertility: is Africa different?', *Lancet* 2, 596–8.
10. Hull, op.cit., p 24.
11. Janice G. Raymond, 'Fetalists and Feminists: they are not the same'. In: Spallone and Steinberg, 1987. See note 2.
12. Mary O'Brien, *The Politics of Reproduction*, Routledge & Kegan Paul, London, 1982.
13. See the arguments made by Jerome Lejeune in, 'Test tube babies *are* babies'. In: *The Question of In Vitro Fertilisation: Studies in Medicine, Law and Ethics*, Evidence to the Government Inquiry into Human Fertilisation and Embryology, from the Society for the Protection of Unborn Children, 1984.
14. John Biggers, Address on the 'Future of human reproduction' to the 1988 meeting of the American Association for the Advancement of Science, Boston.

4. What Goes Wrong? Reproductive Technologies and Infertility

1. Hamish Fraser and J. Waxman, 'Gonadotrophin releasing hormone analogues for gynaecological disorders and infertility'. *British Medical Journal*, 298, 475–6.
2. Pfeffer and Woollett, see chapter 3, note 1, p 12.
3. See Jill Rakusen and Nick Davidson, *Out of Our Hands: What Technology Does to Pregnancy*, Pan, London, 1982, p 108.
4. Ann Oakley, *The Captured Womb*, Blackwell, Oxford, 1984, p 253.
5. Pfeffer and Woollett, see chapter 3, note 1.
6. Jill Rakusen, 'Depo-Provera: the extent of the problem. A case study in the politics of birth control'. In: *Women, Health and Reproduction*, Helen Roberts (ed.), Routledge, London, 1981.
7. Hilary Graham and Ann Oakley, 'Competing ideologies of reproduction: medical and maternal perspectives on pregnancy'. In: Roberts, op.cit., p 66.
8. Italics in original, ibid., p 63.
9. Pfeffer and Woollett, see chapter 3, note 1, p 84.
10. For further discussion of 'success rates' and how they compare with 'normal' pregnancies, see Edward Yoxen, *Unnatural Selection: Coming to Terms with the New Genetics*, Heinemann, London, 1986.

11. Nuala Scarisbrook, quoted by David Fletcher, 'Doctors "stab" three of quins inside womb', *Daily Telegraph*, 21 June 1986.
12. Mary Warnock, *A Question of Life*, The Warnock Report on Human Fertilisation and Embryology, Blackwell, Oxford, 1985, p 36.
13. Elizabeth M. Alder et al., 'Attitudes of women of reproductive age to *in vitro* fertilization and embryo research'. *J. Biosocial Science* 18, 155–67, 1986.

5. Fertilisation and IVF

1. Winston, see chapter 2, note 7, p 152
2. D. Gareth Jones, *Manufacturing Humans*, Intervarsity Press, Leicester, 1987, p 42.
3. Oakley, see chapter 4, note 4, p 283.
4. Gena Corea, *The Mother Machine*, Harper & Row, New York, 1985, p 27.
5. J. Fletcher, The Ethics of Genetic Control, Prometheus Books, New York, 1988.
6. Feminist Self-Insemination Group, *Self Insemination*, PO Box 3, 190 Upper St., London N1, 1980.
7. Renate Duelli Klein, 'Doing it ourselves: self insemination'. In: *Test Tube Women*, Rita Arditti, Renate Duelli Klein and Shelley Minden (eds), Pandora, London, 1984, p 384.
8. Naomi Pfeffer, 'Artificial insemination, in vitro fertilisation and the stigma of infertility'. In Stanworth, see chapter 1, note 17, p 86.
9. Jerome Lejeune, see chapter 3, note 13, p 14.
10. SPUC, *The Question of In Vitro Fertilisation*, 1984, pp 57–8.
11. SPUC, op.cit., 1984, p 59.
12. B. Milbauer, 1983, cited in Janet Gallagher, 'Fetal personhood and women's policy'. In: *Women, Biology and Public Policy*, Virginia Sapiro (ed.), Sage, London, 1985, p 104.
13. Petchesky, *Abortion and Women's Choice*, Verso, London, 1986.
14. Yoxen, see chapter 4, note 10, p 73.
15. Data from the use of GIFT at the Humana Hospital, London: Ian Craft, 'GIFT – the experience of a large United Kingdom series'. In: *Conceive* No. 7. Published by Serono Laboratories, UK, 1987.
16. Lesley Doyal, 'Infertility – a life sentence? Women and the National Health Service'. In: Stanworth, see chapter 1, note 17, 1987.

17. Data compiled from 1985–1987 for a sample of American clinics: Chris Ann Raymond, 'IVF Registry notes more centers, more births, slightly improved odds'. *Journal of the American Medical Association*. 259, pp 1920–1921, 1988.
18. Ibid, pp 1920–21.

6. What Can Go Wrong? Implantation and Pregnancy

1. Pfeffer and Woollett, see chapter 3, note 1, p 110.
2. Oakley, see chapter 4, note 4, p 292.
3. Winston, see chapter 2, note 7, p 55.
4. R. G. Edwards, 'Normal and abnormal implantation in the human uterus', In: *Implantation of the Human Embryo*, R. G. Edwards, J. M. Purdy and P. C. Steptoe (eds), Academic Press, London, 1985.
5. See *Human Embryo Research: Yes or No?*, The Ciba Foundation, Tavistock Publications, London; 1986.
6. Warnock, see chapter 4, note 12, pp 66–67.
7. Ibid., p 91.
8. SPUC, see chapter 5, note 10, p 67.
9. Spallone and Steinberg, Introduction to *Made to Order*, see chapter 3, note 2, p 15.
10. R. G. Edwards, In: *Human Embryo Research*, op.cit., p 142.
11. Sir Cecil Clothier, ibid., p 142.
12. Juliette Zipper and Selma Sevenhuijsen, 'Surrogacy: feminist notion of motherhood reconsidered'. In: Stanworth, see chapter 1, note 17, 1987.
13. Ibid, also see Corea, see chapter 5, note 4, pp 213–49.
14. Our emphasis; SPUC, see chapter 5, note 11, p 70.
15. For detailed discussion of feminist critiques, see Corea, 1985, op.cit. and Christine Overall, *Ethics and Human Reproduction*, Allen and Unwin, London, 1987.
16. Janet Gallagher, 'Eggs, embryos and foetuses: anxiety and the law', In: Stanworth, op.cit., 1987.
17. Zipper and Sevenhuijsen, op.cit.
18. Sue Rodmell, 'Prepregnancy care: whose needs count?' In: *The Politics of Health Education*, Routledge & Kegan Paul, London, 1986.
19. Ibid.
20. Gallagher,: In *Women, Biology and Public Policy*, see chapter 5, note 12. 1985, p 107.

21. Gallagher, 1987, op.cit. pp 139–50.
22. Barbara Katz Rothman, *The Tentative Pregnancy*, Viking, New York, 1986.
23. Gallagher, 1985, op.cit.
24. Oakley, see chapter 4, note 4, p 249.

7. Detecting Genetic Diseases: Prenatal Screening and its Problems

1. Daniel J. Kevles, *In the Name of Eugenics*, Penguin Books, 1986.
2. Mary Sellers, 'Vitamin supplementation and prevention of neural tube defects, In: Gerald Mizejewski and Ian Porter, eds., *Alpha-Fetoprotein and Congenital Disorders*, Academic Press, London, 1985. And Mary Seller, 'Unanswered questions on neural tube defects', *British Medical Journal*, 1987, vol 294, pp 1–2.
3. Stuart Campbell and J. M. Pearce, 'Ultrasound visualisation of congenital malformations', In: *British Medical Bulletin*, 1983, vol 39, pp 322–1. M. d'A Crawfurd, 'Prenatal diagnosis of common genetic disorders', *British Medical Journal*, 1988, vol 297, pp 502–6.
4. Sherman Elias and George J. Annas, 'Routine prenatal genetic screening', *The New England Journal of Medicine*, 1987, vol 317, pp 1407–9.
5. M. S. DiMaio, A. Baumgarten, R. M. Greenstein, H. M. Saul, M. J. Mahoney, 'Screening for fetal Down's syndrome in pregnancy by measuring maternal serum alpha-fetoprotein levels', *The New England Journal of Medicine*, 1987, vol 317, pp 342–6.
6. S. M. Pueschel, 'Maternal alpha-fetoprotein screening for Down's syndrome', *The New England Journal of Medicine*, 1987, vol 317, pp 376–8.
7. Howard Cuckle, 'Screening for fetal and genetic abnormality', King's Fund Forum, London, 30 November to 2 December 1987. King's Fund Centre, 126 Albert Street, London NW1 7.
8. Robert Steinbrook, 'In California, voluntary mass prenatal screening', *Hastings Center Report*, October 1986, p 5. Also op.cit. note 4.
9. R. H. T. Ward, 'Obstetric outcome and problems of midtrimester fetal blood sampling for antenatal diagnosis,' *British Journal of Obstetrics and Gynaecology*, 1981, vol 188, pp 1073–80.

10. For example, Alexander MacLeod and Karol Sikora, eds., *Molecular Biology and Human Disease*, Blackwell Scientific Publications, 1984.
11. Alan Emery, *An Introduction to Recombinant DNA*, John Wiley and Sons, Chichester, 1984.
12. Ibid.
13. Laird Jackson, 'Prenatal genetic diagnosis by chorionic villus sampling', In: Ian Porter, Norma Hatcher, and Ann Willey, eds., *Perinatal Genetics: Diagnosis and Treatment*, Academic Press, 1986.
14. The Ciba Foundation, *Human Embryo Research, Yes or No?*, Tavistock Publications, London, 1986.
15. Nico Leschot, et al, 'Chorionic villi sampling: cytogenetic and clinical findings in 500 pregnancies', *British Medical Journal*, 1987, vol 295, pp 407–10.
16. C. Williams et al, 'Same-day first-trimester antenatal diagnosis for cystic fibrosis by gene amplification', *The Lancet*, 1988, ii, pp 102–3.
17. K. H. Nicolaides, et al. 'Why confine chorionic villus (placental) biopsy to the first trimester?' *The Lancet*, 1986, i, pp 543–4.
18. David Weatherall, *The 'New Genetics' and Clinical Practice*, Oxford University Press, 1985.
19. Stuart Campbell, Department of Obstetrics, King's College, London, personal communication.
20. C. M. Gosden, 'The recognition of clinically significant chromosome abnormalities in prenatal diagnosis: problem cases,' In: C. H. Rodeck and K. H. Nicolaides, eds., *Prenatal Diagnosis*, 1984, Royal College of Obstetricians and Gynaecologists, London.
21. David Weatherall, op.cit., p 182.
22. Wendy Farrant, 'Who's for amniocentesis? The politics of prenatal screening', In: Hilary Homans, ed., *The Sexual Politics of Reproduction*, Gower, Aldershot, 1985.
23. Sally Macintyre, 'Women's experiences and attitudes to screening', In: Screening for fetal and genetic abnormality, King's Fund Forum, see reference 7.
24. *The Lancet*, 26 July 1986, p 225.
25. Bernadette Modell, University College, London, on BBC Horizon programme on the ethics of clinical trials, November 1987.
26. Barbara Katz Rothman, *The Tentative Pregnancy*, Viking, New York, 1986.

27. Bryan Hibbard, 'An obstetric view of population screening programmes', in King's Fund Forum, see reference 7.
28. David Weatherall, op cit.
29. Barbara Katz Rothman, op cit.
30. Edward Yoxen, *Unnatural Selection? Coming to Terms with the New Genetics*, William Heinemann, 1986, p 124.
31. Charles Rodeck, King's College Hospital, London, personal communication.
32. Wendy Farrant, op cit.
33. Peter Harper, 'Genetic counselling and prenatal diagnosis', In: *British Medical Bulletin*, 1983 vol 39, pp 302–09.
34. Anne Finger, 'Claiming all of our bodies', In: *Test Tube Women*, Pandora Press, London, 1984, pp 281–297.
35. Support After Termination For Abnormality (SATFA), National Office, 22 Upper Woburn Place, London WC1H OEP.
36. I. S. Fentiman, 'Pensive women, painful vigils: consequences of delay in assessment of mammographic abnormalities', *The Lancet*, 7 May 1988, pp 1041–2.
37. Viola Roggencamp, 'Abortions of a special kind: male sex selection in India', In: *Test Tube Women*, Pandora Press, London, 1984, pp 266–78.
38. David Weatherall, op cit.
39. Gregory Meissen et al, 'Predictive testing for Huntington's disease with use of a linked DNA marker,' *The New England Journal of Medicine*, 1988, vol 318, pp 535–42.
40. For example, Gina Kolata, 'Manic-Depression: is it inherited?', *Science*, 1986, vol 232, pp 575–6.
41. Bernadette Modell, University College, London, personal communication. See also 'Screening for carriers of recessive disease', in E. O. Carter, ed, *Developments in Human Reproduction and their Eugenic and Ethical Implications*, Academic Press, 1983.
42. Edward Yoxen, op cit. p 119.
43. M. A. Ferguson-Smith, 'Pre-natal chromosome analysis and its impact on the birth incidence of chromosome disorders', *British Medical Journal*, 1983, no. 4, pp 355–64.
44. David Weatherall, op cit.
45. Patricia Spallone and Deborah Lynn Steinberg, eds., *Made to Order*, Pergamon Press, p 6.
46. Edward Yoxen, op cit, p 164.
47. Ian Franklin, 'Services for sickle cell disease: unified approach needed', *British Medical Journal*, 1988, vol 296, p 592. Mary Horn

et al, 'Neonatal screening for sickle cell diseases in Camberwell: results and recommendations of a two year pilot study', *British Medical Journal*, 1986, vol 292, pp 737–40. National Institutes of Health Consensus Conference, 'Newborn screening for sickle cell disease and other hemoglobinopathies,' *Journal of the American Medical Association*, 1987, vol 258, pp 1205–9. Janet Black and Sophie Laws, *Living with Sickle Cell Disease*, East London Branch of the Sickle Cell Society, 1986.
48. Anne McLaren, 'Can we diagnose genetic disease in pre-embryos?', *New Scientist*, 10 December 1987.
49. Edward Yoxen, op cit, p 148.
50. See also Erwin Chargaff, 'Engineering a molecular nightmare,' *Nature*, 1987, vol 327, pp 199–200.
51. Ruth Hubbard, 'Personal courage is not enough', In: *Test Tube Women*, Pandora Press, London, 1984. And Ruth Hubbard, 'Eugenics and prenatal testing', *International Journal of Health Services*, 1986, vol 16, pp 227–42.
52. Eve Nichols, *Human Gene Therapy*, Harvard University Press, 1988.
53. C. Smith et al, *Exploiting New Technologies in Animal Breeding: Genetic Developments*, Oxford University Press, 1986.
54. Edward Yoxen, op cit, p 171.
55. Patricia Spallone and Deborah Lynn Steinberg, eds., *Made to Order*, Pergamon Press, 1986, p 6.
56. Edward Yoxen, op cit, p 119.

8. Towards a Reproductive Future?

1. Peter Singer and Deanne Wells, *The Reproduction Revolution*, Oxford University Press, 1984. pp 131–49.
2. David James, 'Ectogenesis: a reply to Singer and Wells', *Bioethics* 1, pp 80–99, 1987.
3. Robyn Rowland, 'Of Women Born, but for How Long?' In: *Made to Order*, Patricia Spallone and Deborah Lynn Steinberg (eds), Pergamon, 1987, p 77.
4. Anne McLaren, 'Reproductive options, present and future'. In: *Reproduction in Mammals* Book V. *Manipulating Reproduction*, C. R. Austin and R. V. Short (eds), Cambridge University Press, 1986, p 190.
5. J. Fletcher, *The Ethics of Genetic Control*, Doubleday, New York, 1974, pp 147–87.

6. Lejeune, Ramsay and Wright, *The Question of In Vitro Fertilization* op.cit., 1984, p 71.
7. Jeremy Cherfas & John Gribbin, *The Redundant Male*, Paladin, London, 1984.
8. Leon Kass, see chapter 2, note 2.
9. Gena Corea, see chapter 5, note 4, p 80.
10. Ibid., p 39.
11. Ibid., p 46.
12. Ibid., p 280.
13. Margaret Atwood, *The Handmaid's Tale*, Virago, London, 1987.
14. Mary O'Brien, *The Politics of Reproduction*, Routledge & Kegan Paul, London, 1981, p 21.
15. Corea, op.cit., p 289.
16. O'Brien, op.cit., p 22.
17. Feminists have often noted the various meanings of the term 'patriarchy'; see, for instance, Veronica Beechey, 'On patriarchy', *Feminist Review*, 3,66–82, 1979.
18. See, for instance, Jalna Hanmer and Pat Allen, 'Reproductive engineering: the final solution'. In: *Alice Through the Microscope*, Virago, London, 1980: and Helen B. Holmes and Betty B. Hoskins, 'Prenatal and preconception sex choice technologies: a path to femicide?', In: *Man-Made Women*, Gena Corea et al., Hutchinson, London, 1985.
19. Mary Anne Warren, *Gendercide: The Implications of Sex Selection*, Rowman and Allanheld, New Jersey, 1985, pp 173–5.
20. Ibid., pp 163–71.
21. Ibid., pp 175–7.
22. Ibid., pp 176–7.
23. Helen B. Holmes, Review of Warren (op.cit.), *Bioethics* 1, 1987, p 108.
24. Editorial in *British Journal of Sexual Medicine* 10, 14, 1983.
25. Oakley, see chapter 4, note 4.

9. Official Attitudes to Reproductive Technologies in Britain and Elsewhere

1. *The Scientist*, 6 April 1987, p 6.
2. L. Abse, 'The politics of in vitro fertilisation in Britain' in S. Fishel and E. M. Symonds (eds), *In Vitro fertilisation: past, present and future*, IRL Press, Oxford, 1986.

Notes 329

3. *The Australian*, 21 May 86, p 10, reporting on a conference held in Canberra, May 1986, entitled 'Liberation or Loss? Women Act on the New Reproductive Technologies.'
4. See, for example, 'Reproductive Laws for the 1990s: Briefing Handbook' (mimeo), a project cosponsored by the Women's Rights Litigation Clinic and the Institute for Research on Women, Rutgers University, New Jersey.
5. But the tide is turning. In July 1989, a more conservative Supreme Court ruled that individual states could legislate against abortion. However, the Court did not consider whether to overthrow its earlier ruling, upon which women's abortion rights had been based, that the constitutional right to privacy applied to the abortion decision. But this may still come and women's abortion rights in the US are under much greater threat now than at any time in the past twenty years.
6. There are two versions of the Warnock Report. The official version is the *Report of the Committee of Inquiry into Human Fertilisation and Embryology*, Cmnd 9314, HMSO, London, 1984. It was then reissued as a commercial paperback, Mary Warnock, *A Question of Life*, Blackwell, Oxford, 1985 together with two new chapters written by the chairperson on the role of philosophy in policy-making. All subsequent references in this chapter are to the latter version.
7. Study carried out by LeRoy Walters, Director of the Center for Bioethics, Georgetown University.
8. *Human Fertilisation and Embriology: A Framework for Legislation*, Cm 259, HMSO, London, 1987.
9. *Guardian*, 12 August 1988.
10. *The First Report of the Voluntary Licensing Authority for Human In Vitro Fertilisation and Embryology*, Medical Research Council, London, 1986.
11. *Evening Standard*, 19 August 1987.
12. *The Second Report of the Voluntary Licensing Authority for Human In Vitro Fertilisation and Embryology*, Medical Research Council, London, 1987.
13. Warnock, op. cit., p 5.
14. M. Simms, 'Legal abortion in Great Britain' in H. Homans (ed.) *The Sexual Politics of Reproduction*, Gower, Aldershot, 1985, p 79.
15. *On the state of the public health: Annual report to the Chief Medical Officer of the Ministry of Health*, HMSO, London, 1933.
16. Simms, op.cit., p 81.

17. Office of Population Censuses and Surveys, *Abortion Statistics: England and Wales*, HMSO, London, 1986, p 5.
18. Simms, op. cit., pp 94–5.
19. Office of Population Censuses and Surveys, op. cit., p vi.
20. *Women's Reproductive Rights Information Centre Newsletter* July-September 1987, p 3.
21. Lesley Dike, *Late Abortions and Fetal Abnormality*, mimeo, Women's Reproductive Rights Information Centre, London, 1985.
22. Office of Population Censuses and Surveys, *Abortion Statistics: England and Wales*, HMSO, London, 1986, p 5 and OPCS Monitor, AB 87/6, HMSO, London, 1987.
23. *Report of the Select Committee on the Infant Life (Preservation) Bill [H.L.]*, (HL 50), HMSO, London, 1988.
24. Simms, op.cit., p 95.
25. *Guardian*, 6 November 1985.
26. *Sunday Times*, 11 May 1986 and 18 May 1986.
27. *Evening Standard*, 19 August 1987.
28. Gena Corea, see chapter 5, note 4, p 35.
29. Judgement given in Orford v Orford, Supreme Court of Ontario. Although this judgement was typical of many of the time, some British courts ruled differently. It was only finally resolved in Britain in 1959 when MacLennan v MacLennan S.C. 105 established that AID does not constitute adultery. Corea op. cit., p 39.
30. *Sunday Despatch*, 21 November 1945, cited in N. Pfeffer, 'Artificial Insemination, In Vitro Fertilization and the Stigma of Infertility' in M. Stanworth (ed.) *Reproductive Technologies: Gender, Motherhood and Medicine*, Polity Press, Cambridge, 1987, p 93.
31. Ibid, p 92.
32. *Report of the Departmental Committee on Human Artificial Insemination* (Feversham Committee), Cmnd 1105, HMSO, London, 1960.
33. Ibid, p 66, cited in Pfeffer, op. cit., p 94.
34. Law Commission, *Family Law: Illegitimacy*, Working Paper No. 74, HMSO, London, 1982.
35. Warnock, op. cit., p 25.
36. Ibid, p 25.
37. *Human Fertilisation and Embryology*, op.cit., p 14.
38. The Rios case was finally resolved only in 1987 when it was

decided that the embryos could be donated to other infertile couples, but that they would not be entitled to inherit from their genetic parents, *Women's Health and Reproductive Rights Information Centre Newsletter*, No. 1, June 1988, p 11.
39. Warnock, op. cit., p 56.
40. Ibid, p 2.
41. Ibid, p 47.
42. *Human Fertilisation and Embryology*, op.cit., p 12.
43. *Guardian*, 10 January 1987, 12 March 1987, 13 March 1987 and 2 April 1987.
44. Warnock, op. cit., p 47.
45. *Nature*, 15 October 87, p 577.
46. Walters Report, see chapter 9, note 7.
47. *Observer*, 5 April 1987.
48. *Women's Reproductive Rights Information Centre Newsletter*, July-September, 1987.
49. Warnock, op. cit., pp 87–9.
50. Ibid, p 46.
51. Ibid, p xvi.
52. Ibid, p 66.
53. Ibid, p 94. This position is similar to that taken in many other countries. For example, the State of Victoria prohibits research except on spare embryos.
54. Ibid, pp 90–93.
55. *Guardian*, 20 November 1985.
56. Several women's groups gave evidence to the Warnock Committee, including the National Abortion Campaign, Maternity Alliance and Rights of Women.
57. Robyn Rowland, 'Making women visible in the embryo experimentation debate' in *Bioethics*, vol. 1, no. 2, April, 1987.
58. Warnock, op. cit., p 12.
59. Ibid, p 12.
60. Ibid, p 11.
61. *Human Fertilisation and Embryology*, op.cit., p 11.

Conclusion: Policy and Politics

1. Mary Warnock, *A Question of Life*, Blackwell, Oxford, 1985, pp viii, ix.
2. Warnock, Ibid, pp ix–x.

3. Alena Heitlinger, *Reproduction, Medicine and the Socialist State*, Macmillan, Basingstoke, 1987, p 272.
4. Petchesky, *Abortion and Women's Choice*, Verso, London, 1986, pp 346–7.
5. C. Gould, 'Private rights and public virtues: women, the family and democracy' in C. Gould (ed.) *Beyond Domination: New Perspectives on Women and Philosophy*, Rowman and Allanheld, Totowa, New Jersey, 1984, pp 14–15.
6. In 1985, the perinatal mortality rate of babies whose father was of social class I, professional occupations, was 7.8 per thousand live and stillbirths, while for babies whose father was of social class V, unskilled occupations, it was 12.4 per thousand: Office of Population Censuses and Surveys, *OPCS Monitor*, DH3 87/3, p 5.
7. Robyn Rowland, 'Making women visible in the embryo experimentation debate', *Bioethics*, vol. 1, no. 2, 1987, pp 180–3.
8. For discussion of animal experimentation in relation to feminism and science, see Lynda Birke, *Women, Feminism and Biology*, Wheatsheaf, Brighton, 1986.
9. Warnock, op. cit., p 65.
10. Rowland, op.cit., pp 186–7.
11. IVF Australia, set up by the Monash University IVF team, is the most blatant of these companies, see Chapter 2, but this reservation also applies to some extent to all private clinics that do research.
12. Rowland, op.cit., p 180.
13. E. Yoxen, *Unnatural Selection? Coming to terms with the new genetics*, Heinemann, London, 1986, p 29.
14. Small IVF centres, those attempting less than 100 treatment cycles per year, currently give a woman coming for treatment only a 3 per cent chance of giving birth to a live baby as opposed to 20 per cent at the larger centres: *The Third Report of the Voluntary Licensing Authority for Human In Vitro Fertilisation and Embryology*, Medical Research Council, London, 1988.
15. Yoxen, op.cit., p 94.

Index

abortion: access to, 35; anti-abortion lobby, 236–7; for congenital defects, 4, 21, 22–3, 40, 53, 157, 164, 182, 187–8, 291; feminist position, 6–7; illegal, 240–1; late abortions, 245–7; legislation, 233, 240–8; as murder, 73, 118; risks, 27; and sex of child, 21–2, 24, 248; thalidomide cases, 241; women's right to choose, 1–2, 20-2
Abortion Act (1967), 1, 162, 233, 242–7, 248, 271
Abortion Law Reform Association, 244
access to treatment, 35–41, 274–81, 304–6
adoption, 4, 34, 78, 149, 207, 261–2, 264, 301, 308–9
Agricultural and Food Research Council, 221
agriculture; egg harvesting, 220–3; embryo flushing, 138, 220; hybrids, 216–17; transgenic animals, 199
AID *see* artificial insemination by donor
AIDS, 189, 214, 300
AIH *see* artificial insemination by husband
Alder, Elizabeth, 100
alpha fetoprotein (AFP), 166–9, 170, 177, 182, 292
alpha-antitrypsin deficiency, 173
Alton, David, 245–6
Alzheimer's disease, 173, 189
American College of Obstetricians and Gynecologists, 168–9
amniocentesis: and abortion, 27; access to, 40, 163; alpha fetoprotein testing, 166; compared with CVS, 176, 177, 180–1; costs, 163–4; neural tube defects, 164–6; risk of miscarriage, 163; screening for Down's syndrome, 162–4; sex screening, 21–2, 24, 187; timing, 164, 176
anaemia, 191; *see also* thalassaemia, *see also* sickle cell disease
anencephaly, 167, 170
animals: cosmetics testing, 296; egg harvesting, 220–3; embryo flushing, 138, 220; human-animal hybrids, 214–15, 216–17, 229; transgenic, 198–9
antibiotics, 108, 109
antibodies, 106, 108
Aristotle, 68, 69
Arthur, Leonard, 247
artificial insemination, 92, 106–15, 248–55; by donor (AID), 110–14, 248–55, 257, 259, 263, 265, 276, 311; by husband (AIH), 255; self-insemination, 114–15, 254
Australia, 192, 236, 257–8, 273

'Baby M', 264
beta thalassaemia, 173, 191, 193
Biggers, John, 71–2
'biochemical pregnancies', 143–4
Black, Janet, 64–5
black people: access to treatment, 41, 304; black fertility as a problem, 2; genetic screening, 190
blood tests, 166–8, 193, 195
blood transfusion service, 299–300
British Medical Association, 28

British Medical Journal, 178, 249
British Pregnancy Advisory Service, 254–5
Brock, David, 164
buserelin, 90–1, 92

caesarian section, 152–3, 293
capitalism, 30, 47, 55, 229, 251
Catholic Church, 44, 110, 191, 192, 242, 243, 250, 269
cattle, egg harvesting, 138, 220–3
cells, cloning, 211–14
Centre d'Études et de Conservation de Sperme (CECOS), 300
cervix: chorinic villus sampling, 176, 177, embryo transfer, 138
charities: abortion clinics, 243; genetic disease research, 183–4
child-rearing, 307, 312
children: gender stereotyping, 25; 'perfect', 184, 205; role-models, 17, *see also* embryos; fetus
Children's Act (1975), 260, 261, 276
China, 24, 36, 175
choice: and rationality, 26–30; right of, 1–2, 20–5
chorionic villus sampling (CVS), 170, 173–8, 180–1, 187, 196, 197
Christian Action Research and Education Trust, 112
chromosomes, 72, 158; abnormalities, 134, 136, 157–61, 165–6, 177–8; after fertilisation, 106; genetic diseases, 171–2; parthenogenesis, 217, 218
Church of England, 250
Clarke, Tom, 272
clinics: abortion, 242, 243–4, 246, 248; access to, 278, 305–6; artificial insemination, 254
clomiphene, 84, 89, 92, 95, 141, 142
cloning, 205, 210–214, 219–20, 228, 238, 269
Cockburn, Cynthia, 52
Commission on bioethics (USA), 234
Comittee for Abortion Rights and Against Sterilisation Abuse (USA), 3
conception *see* fertilisation
congenital defects: and abortion, 4, 21, 22–3, 40, 157, 164, 182, 187–8, 291; prenatal diagnosis, 4, 21, 23–4, 53, 63, 157–201, 291
Conservative Party, 23–4, 242

contraception, 224–5; Catholic objections to, 44; and choice, 26; injectable, 2, 95; research, 61, 62
contraceptive pills, 61, 155, 225
contracts, surrogacy, 264, 312–13
Corea, Gena, 113, 195, 220–2, 224, 225
Cotton, Kim, 261
counselling: donation, 299, 301; genetic, 79, 185–7, 304; infertility, 279–80, 290–1, 305, 310–11; prenatal diagnosis, 292
Craft, Ian, 239–40
Crowe, Christine, 64
Cuckle, Howard, 168
Cyprus, 192–3
cystic fibrosis (CF), 114, 159, 160, 164, 171–2, 173, 174, 183, 187, 199, 304
cytogenetics, 161–2, 165–6

death: femicide, 226; illegal abortion, 241; mortality, 161, 294; infanticide, 24, 198
Department of Health and Social Security (DHSS), 242, 248
Depo-Provera, 95
diabetes, 174–5
The Dialectic of Sex (Firestone), 43–4
diethylstilboestrol (DES), 96–7
disabled: access to treatment, 41, 64, 247–8, 304; and artificial insemination, 114; society's attitudes towards, 24, 184, *see also* congenital defects
divorce, 32–3, 249, 250
DNA, 72, 158, 160, 171, 172–3, 176, 183, 188, 191–3, 194, 213
doctors *see* medical profession
donors: anonymity, 301, *see also* artificial insemination; eggs, donation
Down's syndrome, 21, 22, 136, 157, 159, 160, 161–4, 168–9, 170, 176, 180, 181–2, 185, 187–8, 190–2
drugs: 'fertility', 77, 85, 91–2; and fetal development, 150; hormonal, 83–4, 88–97, 101; illegal drugs in pregnancy, 153; thalidomide, 241
Duchenne muscular dystrophy, 159, 161, 173, 195–6
Dworkin, Andrea, 220

ectogenesis, 151, 205, 206–10, 219–20, 228, 269, 294

Index

ectopic pregnancy, 89, 91, 98–9, 109, 134, 137, 142–3
Edinburgh, 100, 164, 166, 199
Edwards, R. G., 146, 272
eggs: cloning, 211, 212; division, 106; donation, 33–4, 85, 86, 92, 99–102, 137, 146, 147–9, 255–7, 299–301; failure of fertilisation, 80, 108; fertilisation, 103, 104–6; germline gene therapy, 198–9; GIFT, 122, 123, 126; harvesting, 220–3; human-animal hybrids, 214–215; implantation, 103–4, 130–7; insufficient, 79, 82–3; IVF, 116, 117, 118, 120, 123; multiple pregnancies, 97–8; ownership of, 298–9; parthenogenesis, 215–19; POST, 107, 122, 123; and primacy of male seed, 68, 69; production of, 85–8; retrieval, 94; surrogacy, 262; transport to womb, 107–8
embryos: beginning of life, 295; cloning, 238; development, 69–71; donation, 33–4, 147–9; ectogenesis, 206–10; effects of hormones on, 141–2; embryo flushing, 138, 220; embryo transfer (ET), 81, 137–44, 155; epigenesis, 69; feminist principles, 293–9; freezing, 118, 137, 140–1, 148, 257–8; genes, 71–3; genetic screening, 196–8; human potential, 70–1, 73; hybrids, 216–17; implantation, 70, 130–7; IVF, 104, 117–20, 123–4, 128, 137; legislation, 257–8, 267–74; miscarriage, 80–1, 130–5, 136; moral status, 67, 118–20, 145–6; ownership of, 146–7, 274, 298–9; parthenogenesis, 215–19; preformationism, 69; research, 28, 49, 67, 70, 73, 144–7, 234, 238–9, 267–74, 294–8; sex selection, 248; surrogacy, 262, see also fetus
endocrinology, 61
endometriosis, 108, 109
epidural anaesthesia, 125
epigenesis, 69
ethics, prenatal diagnosis, 178–94
eugenics, 53, 112, 113, 190, 196, 197–8, 205, 246, 249, 295
The Experience of Infertility (Pfeffer and Woollett), 62

FACT (Fertility Action Campaign for Treatment), 63
Fallopian tubes, 86; blockages, 51, 78, 80, 109; ectopic pregnancy, 89, 137, 142; pelvic inflammatory disease, 142; transport of eggs, 107–8
families: artificial insemination, and, 251–3; changing structure of, 32–3; oppressive relations within, 34–5; privacy, 30–2; role of state, 285–6
Family Law Reform Act (1987), 253
farming women, 220–3, 228
Farrant, Wendy, 179
fatherhood, 111–13, *see also* men
femicide, 226
Feminist International Network of Resistance to Reproductive and Genetic Engineering (FINRRAGE), 156
Feminist Self-Insemination group, 115
fertilisation, 104–6; as beginning of life, 71, 72, 103; failure of, 79–80, 104–6, 108–9; human-animal hybrids, 214–15, 216; intervention in, 77; IVF, 103–4, 115–29
'fertility' drugs, 77, 85, 91–2
fetoscopy, 169
fetus: beginning of life, 71–2, 103; chromosome analysis, 161–2, 165; control of its environment, 151; donation, 300; ectogenesis, 151, 206–10; ectopic pregnancy, 142; exposure to hormones, 96–7; feminist principles, 293–9; formation of organs, 150; miscarriage, 80–1; monitoring, 125, 153; moral status, 67; 'mosaic', 177–8; multiple pregnancies, 98–9; photographs of, 120, 150–1; prenatal diagnosis, 157–201; rights, 73, 294; 'selective reduction', 98, 284; sex, 187, 226–7; still-birth, 81; surgery, 153–4; ultrasound scanning, 170, *see also* embryos
Feversham Committee on Human Artificial Insemination, 250–3, 263, 265
Finger, Anne, 186
Firestone, Shulamith, 43–4, 206
Fisher, Geoffrey, Archbishop of Canterbury, 250
Fletcher, Joseph, 114

Food and Drug Administration (FDA), 194
France, 111, 263, 300
frozen embryos, 118, 137, 140–1, 148, 257–8

Gallagher, Janet, 149, 152–3
gametes, 123–4, 257–8, *see also* eggs; sperm
genes, 71–3, 120, 157–9; cloning, 210–14; functions, 121; gene probes, 173, 194; gene therapy, 198–200; parthenogenesis, 218; sex chromosomes, 160–1
genetic counselling, 79, 185–7, 304
genetic disease, 159, 174–5; abortion and, 53; and artificial insemination, 311; in the future, 194–9; gene therapy, 198–9; miscarriage, 134, 136; research, 183–4, 315; screening for, 24, 169–73, 176, 194–9; stillbirth, 81
genetics: and artificial insemination, 113; chromosome analysis, 161–2; and embryo donations, 148, 149; mutations, 160, 174, 195, 213; and parenting, 34, 309, 310
germline gene theapy, 198–200
GIFT (Gamete Intra Fallopian Transfer), 88, 94, 122, 123, 124, 126, 128
Gillick, Victoria, 32
GnRH (Gonadotrophin Releasing Hormone), 90–1
gonadotrophins, 84, 86, 89, 90–1, 92–3
Graham, Hilary, 96
gynaecologists, 50, 55, 279

haemoglobin, 173, 191, 193
haemophilia, 159, 161, 173, 183, 195, 199
Halton septuplets, 92
hamster eggs, 214–15, 216
haploid generation, 72
Harvey, William, 68
Hibbard, Bryan, 182
High Court, 261, 277–8
homeopathy, 83
hormones: 'biochemical pregnancies', 143–4; contraceptive pills, 61; and egg production, 85–8; and embryo transfer, 138–9; and implantation, 132, 133; IVF, 116, 117, 140, 141–2; male infertility, 89–90; and miscarriage, 131–4; retrieval of eggs, 94; and the transport of eggs, 108; treatment of infertility, 83–4, 88–97, 101
House of Commons, 245, 271
House of Lords, 246–7
Hubbard, Ruth, 197
human-animal hybrids, 214–15, 216–17, 229
Humana Hospital, 239–40
Huntington's disease, 160, 173, 188–9, 311
hybrids, human-animal, 214–15, 216–17, 229
hydatiform moles, 70, 219
hydrocephaly, 167
hyperstimulation, ovarian, 93

identical twins, 139, 211, 213–14
illigitimacy, 249–53
immune system, 109, 133, 134, 212
implantation, 80, 103–4, 130–7
in vitro fertilisation (IVF), 85–6; access to, 35–9, 64, 277–8, 305–6; 'biochemical pregnancies', 143–4; and choice, 26–7, 64; costs, 126–7; and ectopic pregnancy, 142–3; egg production, 88; embryo donation, 147–9; embryo research, 144–6, 267–8, 273; embryos, 104, 117–20, 123–4, 128, 137–44; fertilisation, 103–4, 115–29; genetic screening, 196–8; hormone treatment, 91, 92, 93, 96–7, 116, 117, 140, 141–2; implantation, 130; multiple pregnancies, 97–9, 139–40; retrieval of eggs, 94, 116; success rate, 122–4, 127–8, 135; and The Unborn Children (Protection) Bill, 270–1
inbreeding, 110, 174
incompetent cervix, 81, 131
India, 21–2, 174, 187, 191
induction of labour, 154, 155
Infant Life Preservation Act (1929), 246–7
infant mortality, 161, 294
infanticide, 24, 198
infertility: access to treatment, 35–9, 64, 274–81, 304–6; causes, 82; and choice, 26–7, 64; counselling, 279–80, 290–1, 305, 310–11; as a

disease, 65; egg donation, 99–103; as failure, 62–3, 78; failure of fertilisation, 104–6; hormone treatment, 83–4, 88–97, 101; incidence of, 65–7; individuals as focus of, 310–11; justification for research, 60, 62; preventive programmes, 303; as a problem for women, 18–20; research into causes of, 50–1; sperm, 89–90
inheritance, 110, 111, 148, 250, 251, 253, 257–8, 259
injectable contraceptives, 2, 95
insemination see artificial insemination
intelligence, and artificial insemination, 113
International Contraception, Abortion and Sterilisation Campaign, 3
intra-uterine devices (IUDs), 142, 225
Italy, 191, 192, 248
IVF see in vitro fertilisation
IVF Australia, 52

Japan, 161, 237

Kass, Leon, 45, 47, 56, 219–20
King's College Hospital, London, 127
Klinefelter's syndrome, 165
Krobo tribe, 178

laboratories, ectogenesis, 206–10
labour, technological management of, 154–5
Labour Party, 1, 242, 271, 272
Lane Committee, 244
laparoscopy, 94, 117, 122
Law Commission, Working Paper on Illegitimacy, 252–3, 254
Laws, Sophie, 64–5
legislation, 232–3; abortion, 240–8; access to treatment, 274–81; artificial insemination, 250–5; egg donation, 255–7; embryo research, 267–74; embryos, 257–8; fetal rights versus mother's, 152–4, 293; pressure groups, 233–5, 236; surrogacy, 259–67; Warnock Committee, 237–40, 285
legitimacy, 249–53
Lejeune, Jerome, 71, 161
lesbians: access to treatment, 39, 41, 64, 276, 278, 304; artificial insemination, 112, 255

Liberal Party, 242
life: beginning of, 71–2, 103, 295; moral status of embryo and fetus, 67, 118–20, 145–6
Macintyre, Sally, 179–80, 185, 187
McLaren, Anne, 209–10, 213–14
Manchester, 277–8
marker genes, 171–2
marriage: and artificial insemination, 249, 250; economic and social factors, 16; remarriage, 32–3; and surrogacy, 265
medical profession: attitudes towards women, 96; and causes of infertility, 82; control of abortion, 244; control of biological processes, 78–9; control over male partner, 125–6; control of who to treat, 232–3, 242; erosion of women's control, 60, 61–2, 73, 279–80; and IVF, 116; motives, 50; patriarchy, 95
Medical Research Council (MRC), 170, 179, 180–1, 237, 239, 272
medicalisation of reproduction, 60–73
Mediterranean countries, 174, 190, 191
men: alienation from reproduction, 223–4; and artificial insemination, 111–13, 252, 253–4; envy of women's childbearing, 52; genetic connection to child, 34, 309, 310; infertility, 82, 88–90, 125–6; insecurity about paternity, 259; patriarchy, 47, 55, 95, 110, 112–13, 125, 206, 221–6, 228, 230, 285; primacy of sperm, 68–9; stepfathers, 252
menopause, 65, 92
menstruation, 131, 133
mental retardation, 161–2
miscarriages: and amniocentesis, 163–4; and chorionic villus sampling, 176; chromosome abnormalities, 136; in early pregnancy, 71, 80–1, 130–5; and fetoscopy, 169; IVF and, 143; and prenatal testing, 180
Mitterand, François, 263
Modell, Bernadette, 189, 192–3
MOET (multiple ovulation and embryo transfer), 138
molecular diagnosis, genetic diseases, 171–3
Monash University, 52

'morning-after' pills, 108
mortality, infant, 161, 294
'mosaic' fetus, 177–8
The Mother Machine (Corea), 113, 220–2
motherhood: decision to become a mother, 14–20; economic and social factors, 16–17; embryo donation, 147–9; feminism and, 8, 14–15; fetal rights versus mother's 67–8, 73, 152–4, 293; mother's behaviour in pregnancy, 151–2; surrogacy and, 148–9
mucus, cervical, 106, 108
multiple pregnancies, 88, 91–2, 97–9, 139–40, 239, 284
muscular dystrophy, 159, 161, 173, 195–6
mutations, genetic, 160, 174, 195, 213
myotonic dystrophy, 173

National Abortion Campaign, 3
National Health Service (NHS), 236; abortions, 243–5, 246; access to treatment, 278, 305; amniocentesis, 40, 163; artificial insemination, 252; IVF programme, 39, 51, 127; prenatal counselling, 292; prenatal screening, 192
National Opinion Polls, 1–2
nervous system, 150, 296
neural tube defects, 150, 159, 164–9, 177, 181, 182

Oakley, Ann, 63–4, 95, 96, 112–13, 135–6, 155–6, 231
O'Brien, Mary, 31, 223–5
obstetricians, 50, 154, 279
oestriol, 168
oestrogen, 84, 92, 108
Offences Against the Person Act (1861), 240, 241
osteogenesis imperfecta, 188
ovaries, 107; egg harvesting, 220–2; egg production, 85–7; hyperstimulation, 93; polycystic ovary disease, 91, 139; retrieval of eggs, 94; ultrasound imaging, 116, 123
ovulation, 65, 78; failure of, 83; hormone treatment, 84, 93
Oxford, 127, 167, 173, 181, 193

parenting, 33–4, 309
Parkinson's disease, 28

parthenogenesis, 205, 215–19
patriarchy, 47, 55, 95, 110, 112–13, 125, 206, 221–6, 228, 230, 285
pelvic inflammatory disease (PID), 51, 142
Pergonal, 84, 221
Petchesky, Ros, 120, 121, 151
Pfeffer, Naomi, 62, 116
pharmaceutical industry, 51, 61
phenylketonuria (PKU), 159, 173
Piercy, Marge, 43, 54
the Pill, 61, 155, 225
pituitary gland, 86–8, 117
placenta, 132, 133, 150, 175–8
Plaid Cymru, 271
polycystic ovary disease, 91, 139
polymerase chain reaction, 176
POST (Peritoneal Ovum-Sperm Transfer), 107, 122, 123, 124, 128
Powell, Enoch, 269–72, 274
pre-embryos, 120–2, 124, 132, 268
pregnancy: 'biochemical pregnancies', 143–4; choice and, 25–6; cultural images, 121; early miscarriage, 80–1; early stages, 150–4; ectopic, 89, 91, 98–9, 109, 134, 137, 142–3; mother's behaviour during, 151–4; multiple, 88, 91–2, 97–9, 139–40, 239, 284; as restriction, 206; surrogacy, 34, 85, 111, 137, 148–9, 206–7, 216, 217, 238, 259–67, 312–13; testing kits, 144
'prenatal adoption', 148, 149
prenatal diagnosis, 157–201; access to, 40–1, 64–5; alpha fetoprotein testing, 166–9, 170, 177, 182, 292; and choice, 26, 27; chorionic villus sampling, 170, 173–8, 180–1, 187, 196, 197; congenital defects, 4, 21, 23–4, 53, 63, 291; embryos, 196–8; ethics, 178–94; feminist principles, 303–4; motives for, 53; risk of miscarriage, 163–4, 169, 176, 180, sex of child, 21, 24–5, 187, 226–7; for thalassaemia, 191–3; women's attitudes to, 179–82, *see also* amniocentesis
pressure groups, 233–5, 236
preventive programmes, 37, 38, 51, 303
progesterone, 108, 132, 138–9, 140
'Progress' campaign, 271–2

'Progress and Humanity' campaign, 272
prostaglandins, 109
prostitution, 220, 266–7
public debate, 313–14

quality control, artificial insemination, 112–13, 115

racism, 183, 190
rape, 235, 241, 278
rationality, and choice, 26–30
recessive genes, 160
Rehibin, 84
Renaissance, 48
The Reproduction Revolution (Singer and Wells), 206
research: egg harvesting, 100; on embryos, 28, 49, 67, 70, 73, 144–7, 234, 238–9, 267–74, 294–8; genetic diseases, 315; into contraception, 61, 62; justification of, 60, 61–4; motives for, 51–4; prenatal diagnosis, 182–4; and profitability, 52
Rhesus babies, 157
Richardson, Jo, 271
'right to choose', 1–2, 20–5
'Rios twins', 258
Rodeck, Charles, 184
Rodmell, Sue, 152
Rothman, Barbara Katz, 26, 153–4, 181–2, 184, 187
Rowland, Robyn, 208
Royal College of Obstetricians and Gynaecologists, 237, 239, 252, 272, 296

San Francisco, 172–3
Sardinia, 191, 192
Scarisbrook, Nuala, 98
schizophrenia, 173, 189
science: control of, 49–50, 315; distrust of, 48; dynamics of, 48–9; feminist responses to, 50–6; moral neutrality, 47, 219; and 'nature', 43–7, 56; and social need, 49
Scotland, 190–2, 248
screening *see* prenatal diagnosis
'selective reduction', 98, 284
self-help groups, 114–15, 186
self-insemination (SI), 114–15, 254, 302
Sevenhuijsen, Selma, 149
sex of child: and abortion, 248; prenatal diagnosis, 21, 24–5, 187, 226–7, 292–3
sex chromosomes, 158, 160–1, 165, 187
Shockley, William, 113
sickle cell disease, 159, 173, 174, 182–3, 187–8, 190, 191, 195, 304, 311
Singer, Peter, 206, 207
single mothers, 33, 276, 278
social need, research and, 61–4
society, and control of science and technology, 49–50
Society for the Protection of Unborn Children (SPUC), 103, 115–18, 145–6, 148, 215
somatic gene therapy, 198, 199–200
sperm: antibodies to, 108–9; artificial insemination, 33–4, 110–14, 248–55, 300–1; assessing quality, 214–15; capacitation, 105; failure of fertilisation, 79–80, 89, 106, 108–9; fertilisation of egg, 103, 104–6; freezing, 257; hormone treatment, 89–90; human-animal hybrids, 214–15, 216; insufficient, 79, 82–3; IVF, 117, 123; ownership of, 298–9; and parthenogenesis, 218–19; POST, 107; primacy of, 68–9; self-insemination, 114–15; sperm banks, 110–111, 112, 114, 300; surrogacy, 262–3
spina bifida, 150, 159, 164, 167, 170, 175, 177, 201
state, role of, 285–7
status quo, 46–7
Statutory Licensing Authority (SLA), 238–9, 255, 260, 265, 268, 269, 277, 279–80, 306
Steel, David, 242
Steptoe, Patrick, 248
sterilisation, 51, 66, 146, 273
still-birth, 81
storage, embryos and gametes, 257–8
stress, 65, 83, 152
Support After Termination for Abnormalities (SATFA), 186
support groups, 114–15, 186
surgery: fetal, 153–4; legal compulsion on women to undergo, 152–4
surrogacy, 34, 85, 111, 137, 148–9, 206–7, 216, 217, 238, 259–67, 312–13

Surrogacy Arrangements Act (1985), 238, 261
Surrogate Parenting Agency, 261

Tay-Sachs disease, 114, 174, 182, 190, 311
The Tentative Pregnancy (Rothman), 181
'test-tube babies', 43; *see also* in vitro fertilisation
Testard, Jacques, 197
Thailand, 191–2
thalassaemia, 65, 159, 173, 174, 176, 183, 188, 189, 190, 191–3, 195, 198, 311
Thalassaemia Society, 197
thalidomide, 96, 150, 241
Thatcher, Margaret, 1
Thurnham, Peter, 271
Trades Union Congress, 1
transgenic animals, 198–9
TUDOR (trans-vesicle, ultrasound directed oocyte recovery), 94
Turner's syndrome, 165
twins, 70, 88, 139, 143, 170, 211, 213–14, 268

ultrasound scanning, 116, 123, 143, 144, 157, 166, 169, 170, 176–7
The Unborn Children (Protection) Bill, 269–72
United States of America; abortion rights, 236–7; access to treatment, 277; AFP-testing, 167–9; artificial insemination, 249; chorionic villus sampling, 175, 176; embryo research, 234; gene therapy, 198; genetic screening, 190; legal intervention against mothers, 152–4; malpractice suits, 233; prenatal counselling, 186, 292; reproductive rights, 3; right-wing attitudes to feminism, 32; sex-selective abortion, 248; surrogacy, 261, 264; withdrawal of treatment from disabled babies, 247
University of Wales College of Medicine, 182
uterus: artificial insemination by donor, 110; in early pregnancy, 151; failure of implantation, 80; implantation of embryo, 70, 130–7; transport of eggs to, 107–8
utilitarianism, 282–4

varicocele, 89
virgin birth, 217
Voluntary Licensing Authority for Human in Vitro Fertilisation and Embryology (VLA), 98, 239, 272

Warnock, Dame Mary, 70, 237
Warnock Committee, 9, 240; access to treatment, 274; artificial insemination, 111, 112, 253–4, 255–7; egg donation, 99–100; embryo research, 70, 145, 267–71, 272, 274; human-animal hybrids, 215; IVF, 120, 148–9; legislation, 234, 238, 285; moral conflicts, 282–3; prenatal diagnosis, 197; proposals, 237–8; storage of gametes and embryos, 258; surrogacy, 148, 260–1, 262–3, 265–6
Warren, Mary Anne, 227
Weatherall, David, 178–9, 192, 193, 194
Wells, Deanne, 206, 207
West Germany, 263–4
White Paper, 238, 256
Whitehead, Mary Beth, 264
Wigley, Dafydd, 271
Winston, Robert, 49
Woman on the Edge of Time (Piercy), 43, 54
womb *see* uterus
'womb-leasing', 148
Women's Global Network on Reproductive Rights, 3
Women's Health and Reproductive Rights Information Centre, 3
Women's Reproductive Rights Campaign, 3, 246
Women's Reproductive Rights Information Centre, 3
Woollet, Anne, 62
World Health Organisation (WHO), 191, 193

X-rays, 170
XYY syndrome, 165–6

York, Archbishop of, 271
Yoxen, Edward, 183, 190, 195, 197, 200–1, 312

Zipper, Juliette, 149
zygotes, 123–4